Living Lessons

Living Lessons

Mark Shigihara, RPh
with Kim Erickson

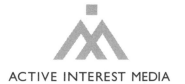

ACTIVE INTEREST MEDIA

Published by:
Active Interest Media, Inc.
300 N. Continental Blvd., Suite 650
El Segundo, CA 90245

Text design by Karen Sperry
Cover design by Silke Design

The information in this book is for educational purposes only and is not recommended as a means of diagnosing or treating an illness. All health matters should be supervised by a qualified healthcare professional. The publisher and the author are not responsible for individuals who choose to self-diagnose and/or self-treat.

Library of Congress Cataloging-in-Publication Data
Shigihara, Mark
Living Lessons / Mark Shigihara with Kim Erickson
Includes bibliographical references and index.
1. Cancer 2. Inspirational 3. Spiritual 4. Integrative Treatment 5. Mind/Body 6. Title

ISSN: 978-1-935297-33-8

Printed in the United States of America

Dedication

To my Gwen, James, and Lane, whose love, prayers,
and unfailing support have inspired me to live.

And, for cancer patients and the people
who love them. Together, we will make
each day our masterpiece.
Mark

☙

For my amazing husband, Mike, who encourages me
to be my best self every day.
Kim

Please Note

Acknowledgments

What a journey it has been . . . and the end
is not in sight.
~ from the song The Journey, Lea Salonga

From Mark

My journey would not have been possible without the amazing support of my family, friends, and coworkers. There are too many of you to recognize individually by name—that would constitute another book. However, please know that you are in our hearts, and our gratitude holds no bounds. This journey of life is thanks to the extraordinary care of many healthcare team members including Dr. Ben Chue, Dr. James Cunningham, Dr. Mika Sinanan, Dr. George Pappas, Dr. Paul Reilly, Dr. Bruce Tung, and my amazing acupuncturist, Darin Bunch.

My hat is off to Kim Erickson. You are an incredible coauthor and I know that patients will benefit from your insights. Thanks to Karolyn Gazella who saw the vision of this journey. Sandy Salzberg—you have been there every step of the way making this dream come true. For my mom, Betty Shigihara—thank you for teaching this dyslexic child to read and write. This book is possible because of your love and devotion. James and Lane, you have been ideal sons whose support has been unwavering. You have made your dad proud. But most of all,

Gwen, you are a beautiful and caring wife who has made my journey and this book a reality.

Finally, thanks to God for giving me the time and strength to write this book and help others.

From Kim

Putting a book together is a massive project involving many people. First and foremost, I would like to thank Mark Shigihara, who was the driving force behind this book. I would also like to thank our publisher, Karolyn Gazella, our editor, Deirdre Shevlin Bell, and the entire team at Active Interest Media for all of their hard work. In addition, I want to express my appreciation to all of the healthcare professionals and Shigihara family members who contributed their wisdom to this project. Finally, a huge thank you to my husband for his unfailing love and support—even when work took precedence over making dinner.

Contents

Foreword xi

Preface xiii

Introduction xv

CHAPTER 1   A Life Before Cancer 1

CHAPTER 2   Testing 1, 2, 3 9

CHAPTER 3   How Did This Happen? 23

CHAPTER 4   So Doc, What Are My Options? 35

CHAPTER 5   A Different Point of View 49

CHAPTER 6   Complementing Chemo 73

CHAPTER 7   A Healthier Way of Living 99

CHAPTER 8   The Advantages of Acupuncture 117

CHAPTER 9   The Mind-Body Connection 131

CHAPTER 10   More than Just Medicine 149

CHAPTER 11   Dealing with Setbacks 159

CHAPTER 12   Caregiving: Caring for Your Loved One,

                     Caring for Yourself 167

APPENDICES   Resources 183

                     Glossary 193

                     Selected References 203

                     Index 215

Foreword

BEING A PHARMACIST AS WELL AS an information technology careerist, it's my life's mission to convey technology innovation in medicine. For that reason, I am honored to introduce *Living Lessons: A Journey of Love, Faith, and Cutting-Edge Cancer Treatment*. Mark Shigihara is not only a cancer patient and a fellow pharmacist, but he has also been a good friend for the past 28 years.

Living Lessons chronicles Mark's experience with pancreatic cancer, a rollercoaster ride full of trepidation, physical and emotional pain, and suffering. Instead of responding to these huge and unknowable adversaries with fear and despair, Mark tackles these challenges with immense courage and grace. He has become the cheerleader—the one who united his family, friends, and colleagues to take this journey together. It is a remarkable journey that glorifies our faith, grows our relationships, and celebrates our lives.

Being a dedicated evidence-based medicine practitioner, Mark saw the opportunity to transform his dreadful journey into a real time, fact-driven, clinical trial on pancreatic cancer using himself as the test subject. He meticulously synthesized his extensive research on a wide range of pancreatic cancer treatment models and methodically described his treatment experience in fine detail for the reader.

Through *Living Lessons*, Mark and his coauthor, Kim Erickson, illustrate how the pancreatic cancer patient can live a full and cherished life with courage and grace under fire. Whether you are a cancer patient or a loved one who takes care of one, you will find this book invaluable in obtaining useful insights and knowledge to help you navigate the road ahead.

Steve T. Chin, RPh
Formerly the Global Life Sciences
Industry Manager
Microsoft Corporation

Preface

THIS ISN'T A BOOK ABOUT DYING. It's a book about living. A book about courage and perseverance. A book about grace under fire.

I first met Mark Shigihara during a conference call with my editor, Karolyn Gazella, and Mark's best friend, Sandy Salzberg. I was actually a bit surprised to find myself on the phone at all. After all, this wasn't a project I really wanted to get involved in. As I told Karolyn, I write books about science and medicine—both conventional and holistic. I am perfectly happy spending my days mired in clinical trials and evaluating the effectiveness of this diet or that supplement. For better or for worse, I'm not the touchy-feely type; I prefer facts over untidy emotions.

My books and articles focus on these facts—and on improving people's wellness by educating them about their healthcare options. So when Karolyn approached me with an opportunity to coauthor a book with someone who had been diagnosed with stage 4 pancreatic cancer, my first inclination was to take a pass. Had I acted on this inclination, I would have missed getting to know a truly remarkable man.

Mark, it turns out, comes from the same fact-based world I do. As a clinically based pharmacist, he spends long hours poring over the latest research. For him to embrace an integrative approach to his cancer treatment was a leap of faith. And yet, this unconventional approach to an aggressive and fatal cancer has earned him time he may not have enjoyed had he relied solely on conventional cancer care. But it wasn't just the novel form of chemotherapy he received, nor the herbs, diet, or acupuncture that extended his life. It was also Mark's faith and attitude that has helped him survive. Mark possesses a rare inner strength and uncomplaining spirit that continually amazes me. Events that would leave most of us quaking do not deter Mark from his ultimate goal of living.

I know a book about cancer may not be the most entertaining of reads. And yet, it is our sincere hope that cancer patients, their caregivers, healthcare providers, and anyone facing a critical challenge in life are able to benefit from the valuable lessons of Mark's own experience.

Cancer changes your life, and sometimes for the better. That may sound strange but, over the course of writing this book with Mark, I have discovered a four-letter word that makes all the difference: Hope. As the early 20th century motivational author, Orison Swett Marden, observed, "There is no medicine like hope, no incentive so great, and no tonic so powerful as the expectation of something tomorrow."

Kim Erickson

Introduction

I T WAS AN UNUSUALLY CALM, DRY December afternoon as I pulled our gold minivan out of the Starbucks parking lot. Just a week before, torrents of rain and howling wind swept through the streets of Bellevue, Wash., ripping at shingles and downing trees. But, today seemed like the calm after the storm.

On any other day, I would be heading home from either working with a University of Washington School of Pharmacy student or a meeting with one of several clients in the pharmaceutical industry. But today was different. Today I was on my way to see the doctor. As I shifted the van into drive, I hoped I could get some answers for the wide array of problems that had plagued me over the past six months—the sinus infection that never went away, frequent colds I simply couldn't shake, nagging gastrointestinal problems. As the months rolled by, I also noticed that my urine was unusually dark and my complexion had taken on a yellow tinge. And then there was the itching that no amount of scratching would relieve.

All of these unrelated signs told me that something was wrong, but I had simply ignored them. After all, I had always been healthy—and between an unrelenting work schedule and the upcoming holidays, I really didn't have time to be sick.

As I drove, I wondered if perhaps my workaholic lifestyle had finally caught up with me. I've been a pharmacist for the past quarter century and, along with providing pharmaceutical education for drug companies, I serve on the affiliate faculties of several colleges and universities. I am also an affiliate assistant professor at the University of

Washington Pharmacy School, specializing in evidence-based medicine review. With all of these career commitments, it wasn't unusual for me to put in 12- to 16-hour days.

What little downtime I did allow myself was spent with my wife and two growing sons, James and Lane. Turning into the doctor's complex, I smiled to myself as I thought of Christmas, just three days away. The tree was trimmed, the presents bought and wrapped. Even though the boys were getting older, the whole family had a sense of seasonal excitement. Now, if the doctor could just figure out what was going on, I could enjoy the holiday with my family and get on with my life.

Yes, it was the calm after the storm—or so I thought. Little did I know that I would soon be confronted with a physical and emotional storm unlike anything I could ever imagine.

*   *   *   *

Cancer is not a death sentence. It is a reaffirmation of life.

I write these words during another Christmas season, three years after that first doctor's appointment. This, in itself, is remarkable. After all, most people diagnosed with stage 4 pancreatic cancer are told they have only weeks or months to live. I have been fighting back—and winning—for *years*. While optimism, perseverance, and faith have played a critical role in staying alive, it was the combination of conventional and unconventional cancer therapies that I credit with my ability to beat the odds.

As an evidence-based pharmacist, I've spent my entire adult life working on behalf of patients to help them understand and adhere to their drug therapy. Much of my career has been devoted to analyzing peer-reviewed drug studies and presenting the data to health plan and government bodies with the hope that appropriate choices will be made for patients. Some of my presentations have influenced drug therapy for millions of patients. With decades of standard "by the book" training, you would think that my automatic knee-jerk reaction to a cancer diagnosis would have been conventional drugs and treatments. But when it's personal, when it's *your* life at stake, you want to know every single option available. This is what led me to broaden my horizons.

Hearing the words "you have cancer" is similar to a sledgehammer smacking you right in the jaw. When the doctor then tells you it is pancreatic cancer—a cancer with incredibly grim survival rates—it feels like the entire world is crashing down around you. Like most people diagnosed with pancreatic cancer, mine wasn't detected until it had spread to my lymph nodes, the ducts leading into the small intestines, and my colon. Unlike some other forms of cancer, like slow-growing thyroid or prostate cancer, this type of cancer spreads easily out of the pancreas because the main function of the pancreas is to produce enzymes and hormones that are pushed out into the bloodstream and digestive system. This means that the cancer cells have easy access to the rest of the body before you even know it exists.

Once the initial shock of my diagnosis and the fear for my family began to ebb, I made a very fundamental decision: I was going to fight this cancer with all my might and not leave any stone unturned. Thanks to my medical background, I knew exactly what I was facing. I was familiar with many of the conventional cancer treatments that were available to people in my position. But I wanted to know what other options were available to treat the cancer itself and help me hang on to my quality of life. While I didn't turn my back on conventional surgery and chemotherapy, I began to embrace the alternatives. Guided by a remarkable medical team that included an integrative oncologist, a naturopath, and an acupuncturist, I opened myself up to the best of all worlds of medicine.

When I chose to pursue an integrative treatment plan, I never intended to downplay the incredible contributions of allopathic medical practitioners who follow traditional cancer protocols. From their perspective, they are following their best judgment and are acting in the best interest of patients. The protocols they rely on have predictable results. And, while treatments like radiation and chemotherapy have well-documented side effects, they *are* proven to kill cancer cells. This is good enough for many doctors and they look no further for alternative treatments. Other physicians simply aren't aware of the vast number of adjunct therapies that can complement or be used in lieu of conventional protocols. Some of these alternatives are treatments most physicians have never heard of. Others may ring a bell, but busy doctors just don't have the time to comb the medical literature in search of proof that this herb or that unconventional treatment can benefit their patients. After all, when you are dealing with devastating cancers such as pancreatic cancer, a patient's time is paramount.

Doctors who only consider a conventional approach aren't alone in missing out on the benefits of complementary medicine. Many patients, faced with the terrifying diagnosis of cancer, go along with whatever their healthcare providers recommend—no questions asked. But taking this path of least resistance, while it may seem easier, may not be the best choice. My own exploration into the alternatives to standard cancer treatment was, in a way, a leap of faith for me. It certainly wasn't what my family, friends, and doctors expected, considering my background. But the rewards of blending the best of both healing options—along with my strong spiritual faith, enduring love of family, and sheer stubbornness—have not only extended the quantity of my life, they have also vastly improved its quality.

At some point in time, my new lease on life will expire, but that should not be a time of sorrow. The sadness will be balanced by the recollection that, while my journey on earth has ended, it was filled with many wonderful memories. It was a life shortened in quantity by cancer but enriched in quality. It has also provided me an opportunity to help others. In the meantime, I am committed to educating and inspiring others living with cancer, as well as their caregivers and loved ones. This book is about faith, hope, perseverance, and knowing your options. It is my hope that sharing my story will, in some small way, help others who face life-altering challenges.

CHAPTER ONE

Life Before Cancer

Other things may change us, but we start
and end with the family.
~ *Anthony Brandt*

I HAVE ALWAYS FELT BLESSED. The youngest of three children—and the only boy—I made my appearance during the sunset of the "Fabulous 1950s." Life seemed simpler in the 50s and early 60s. Some even say it was an idyllic time in American history. After all, World War II was over and jobs were plentiful. The Great Depression was a distant memory. Suburbs sprang up like weeds all over the country and a growing number of families became the proud owners of homes, cars, and television sets. It was a time when families sat around the dinner table together and parents tried to shield their children from the harsh realities of the world around them.

Growing up in this era of peace and prosperity seemed like something right out of a Norman Rockwell painting. When I wasn't doing schoolwork or playing with the neighborhood kids, I would spend my days collecting fossils and poring over comic books. A strong sense of right and wrong, combined with my participation in a variety of sports, kept me from getting into too much mischief.

Rainy days, something Seattle experiences frequently, were spent indoors watching *Leave It to Beaver*, *Lassie*, and *My Three Sons*. To me, these shows were a reflection of my reality. Family was the cornerstone of my existence and, at least to me, father really did know best.

Dad was always my hero. When I was very young, he was the center of my tiny universe. In my mind, Dad could solve any problem, no matter how big, and protect us from any danger, no matter how ominous. Even though he didn't often tell me how much he loved me, my father was always there for me and my sisters, putting our needs before his. As a result, there was never a moment when I didn't feel loved and secure.

As I got older, I learned what a remarkable man he really was. As a young man, my father had dreams of becoming a veterinarian. But his dream was cut short by World War II. While the war interrupted the lives of millions of Americans, it was quite different for those of Japanese descent like my father. Fear gripped America in the wake of the attack on Pearl Harbor. Anyone living in the United States with even a drop of Japanese blood—even those who were U.S. citizens—were suspected of having loyalties to the enemy. On February 19, 1942, President Franklin D. Roosevelt signed Executive Order 9066, which set the stage for establishing internment camps where more than 110,000 Japanese Americans would be confined until the war was over. My father, at the tender age of 20, was one of these people.

With only the possessions they could carry, my father and his family were given just 48 hours to leave their home. They had no idea when, or even if, they would be allowed to return. Once they arrived at Camp Minidoka in Hunt, Idaho, they found conditions in the internment camp poor. The meals were unappetizing and medical care inadequate. The walls in the barracks were insulated with tar paper, and dust crept in through every crack and crevice. There was little privacy, no running water, and no lavatories in the barracks—which meant that people had to make their way to a separate building that housed the laundry and bathrooms, even in the middle of frigid winter nights.

Although most of the interned tried to prove themselves loyal by complying with the U.S. government, there was much bitterness. In spite of this growing resentment, my father's sense of honor and obligation as an American citizen remained strong. As a result, he made the controversial choice to join the military as part of the secret Military Intelligence Service. Over the objections of many of his fellow detainees, my father spent long days stationed in a camouflaged building in Vint Hill, Va., decoding Japanese messages in an attempt to help the war effort and save the lives of American soldiers. For my father, it was simply the right thing to do.

After the internment camps were deemed unconstitutional in 1945, my father's family returned to Seattle. But he would not join them until his discharge from the military in 1947 after serving as an interpreter in occupied Japan. Instead of returning to school, my father decided to join the post-war workforce so that he could help support his mother and youngest brother. He made the same honorable choice on behalf of his wife and family years later when he took a job at Boeing designing airplane cabins. It wasn't his dream job by any stretch of the imagination. In fact, it was a 37-year career filled with stress and anxiety. Yet, in order to provide us with the best life he possibly could, my father gladly got up every morning and went to work. Family was everything to my father, and so it was the right thing to do.

My mother also sacrificed. As a secretary, she was constantly juggling work and family during an era when most women stayed at home to raise their children. Yet, we never felt neglected. In fact, when I was struggling in school, Mom put everything aside to help me manage what we later learned was dyslexia. When I was in the fourth grade, we moved from Seattle to Renton, WA. But instead of forcing me to change schools mid-year, she would wake me up early and drive an extra 30 minutes to drop me off at my old school so that I could complete the school year with my classmates. She also spent many hours helping me with my homework. If not for my mother's efforts, I would never have gone on to college and certainly would never have become a successful pharmacist and educator.

A very spiritual person, my mother always put other people's needs ahead of her own. This was true throughout her life. Mom knew what it was like to be uprooted and displaced. She and her family were also interned at Camp Minidoka—although she didn't meet my father until after the war was over. Her teenage years were spent attending the camp school and working in the canteen. During her family's internment, her father died after a long illness. Her mother, a successful businesswoman before the war, cleaned offices and barracks in the camp. There was little time for fun. My mother was determined that her children would have a better life than she did.

While I got my sense of honor and a solid work ethic from my parents, I developed my sense of fun at the expense of my sisters. Being the youngest, I was always doted on by my sisters, Patti and Terri—at least until I got underfoot. Because I was so much younger than my sisters—Patti is seven years my senior and Terri, five—they were often charged with babysitting. This gave me the perfect opportunity to hone my skills as a prankster.

Being the only boy had its perks, too. As often as he could, Dad would hurry home and we would head out to root for one of our favorite teams—just the two of us. On the way to the game, we would talk about school, family, and my own adventures in whichever sport I was playing at the moment. On the way home, we would relive the game—the spectacular plays, blown calls, and last-second heroics. During these chats, my father would always manage to weave little life lessons into our conversations. While I wasn't always thrilled when the talk turned to the value of hard work, the importance of education, family priorities, and how doing what was right was always better than doing what was popular, these lessons took root in my brain and have stayed with me to this day. They are one reason I am the man I am today.

Unfortunately, the same can be said of our other game-day tradition—those post game stops at a local burger joint. For me, it was always a couple of mega-burgers, a large order of fries, and a vanilla shake. If gluttony is one of the seven deadly sins, I suppose I've always been guilty—especially when it comes to fast food. I've never met a cheeseburger I didn't like and have made them a fixture in my diet. Little did I know that all of that unhealthy fat and sugar would gradually contribute to a life-threatening health crisis years later.

The All-American Dream

By the time I started high school I had pretty much adapted to my learning difficulties—but I still had the feeling that I needed to work harder than my peers. And work, I did. It seemed like I was always studying. In the end, it paid off. I was class valedictorian and graduated with a 4.0 grade point average. When my nose wasn't buried in chemistry and biology books—two of my favorite subjects—I was scrambling to beat deadlines for the school newspaper where I served as the sports editor. Whenever there was any downtime, you could find me searching out a pickup basketball game. Sports have always been my passion. From cheering on the Seattle Supersonics to reporting on Hazen High's football team, I was the ultimate sports fan. I still am.

College life was even more hectic. As a pre-pharmacy student at Seattle University and then a full-fledged pharmacy study at the University of Washington, I soaked up everything I could, managing to make the Dean's list and Rho Chi—the pharmacy school's honor society. I was fortunate to find something I loved and was good at an early age. Not everyone was so lucky. Some of my classmates were really struggling academically, and I found myself working as a tutor. It was a win-win situation. They got help with their studies and I had the opportunity to make a few extra bucks.

I also put in 20 hours a week at Providence Hospital as a pharmacy intern and even managed to play intramural basketball throughout my college years. Looking back, I wonder how I was ever able to squeeze so many activities into so few hours. When you are young, you think you are invincible, but there was a limit—even for me. With everything I had going on, there simply wasn't any time for dating, let alone a relationship. Of course, this didn't stop my friends from trying to set me up.

Shortly before spring in 1981, a friend of mine from the pharmacy school started to pester me about joining him on a double-date. He said there was someone that his girlfriend wanted me to meet. *I really don't have time*, I thought, *and besides, a blind date?* But he was insistent and I finally gave in just to get him off my back. It was the best move I've ever made.

Gwen was graceful and intelligent with a wonderful sense of humor. Now, I had never been one to believe in love at first sight, but I was smitten. The same couldn't be said for Gwen. Like me, she was focusing on her studies. But, unlike me, she wasn't so easily swayed by love. An education major, Gwen had it all figured out: Once she graduated with her teaching degree, she would settle in Hawaii and kick-start her career as a special education teacher. Period.

Gradually, I wore her down and her visions of paradise gave way to the possibility of spending the rest of her life in the damp and gloomy Pacific Northwest. Three and a half years later, Gwen and I were wed. As we settled into married life, I began to climb the corporate ladder at a national pharmaceutical company while Gwen taught students with special needs in Seattle's school district. Our nights were often spent swapping stories about the highlights of the day. While I felt I was performing an important service within the medical community, listening to Gwen recount her day always made me realize just how important her role as an educator really was. Her passion for teaching children with learning, emotional, and behavioral disabilities, as well as health impairments like cerebral palsy, autism, and Down syndrome, was truly inspiring.

In August 1989, we became the happy parents of a baby boy. James turned out to be a colicky baby. All that crying and fussing truly tested our resolve, but after a few short months, James became the best of babies. Even today, he is the most cheerful and optimistic person I know.

Lane followed in June of 1992—a month before his due date. While he didn't suffer from colic, he was hit with a series of severe ear infections that left him with a hearing impairment. While this has been challenging, his sheer determination and competitive spirit have help him overcome any difficulties his hearing loss has posed.

It was a storybook life unmarred by the difficulties my parents had faced. I had a loving family and a good career. We wanted for nothing. While I was an admitted workaholic, family was everything. It truly didn't get any better than this.

Subtle Signs of Something Wrong

This perfect life I had so carefully constructed started to shatter when I began experiencing a series of seemingly unrelated health problems. It began during the summer of 2006 while the family was on vacation in New York City. As we explored the sights and sounds of the Big Apple, I noticed that I was just feeling a little "off." Since I had always been the picture of health, I chalked it up to my body trying to adjust to the difference in time, weather, and food. But the feeling persisted long after the vacation was over.

Autumn descended on the Pacific Northwest and my typical workload increased with the beginning of school. Along with my "day job" as a district manager in the pharmaceutical industry, I also served as an affiliate assistant professor with the University of Washington School of Pharmacy. As such, I would lecture on evidence-based medicine and formulary management. I also routinely met with pharmacy students in their final year at various schools to help them hone the skills they would need in the real world.

As I geared up for the fall semester, I started to develop troublesome colds and sinus infections that I just couldn't shake. Then one night, I fell victim to extreme indigestion and gastrointestinal upset after eating one of my favorite meals—a big platter of deep-fried shellfish with a side of French fries. I momentarily considered going to the doctor to seek relief, but as soon as the symptoms passed, I brushed the incident aside. After all, I didn't have time to be sick!

Of course, these weren't the only clues that something was wrong. A few weeks later, I noticed that my urine was becoming progressively darker—a sign that bilirubin might be accumulating in my bile ducts. Not long after, I began to itch all over. Thinking I had developed an allergy to something Gwen was using, I asked her if she had switched our laundry detergent or had picked up a different brand of bath soap. She hadn't.

What shocked both Gwen and me was the day we saw our reflection in the mirror as we stood side by side. Gwen's coloring was normal, but mine had an odd yellow tinge. If I had been thinking objectively, I would have recognized this as an unmistakable sign that my bile ducts were blocked. However, I just chalked it up to the fluorescent lighting. To be on the safe side, I made a mental note to give the doctor a call. But, between the demands of work and family, I never quite got around to picking up the telephone.

While my appetite was fine, I noticed that I was also having trouble digesting the foods I ate, especially if they were filled with fat. After a meal, I would experience a distinct band of pressure in my abdominal area. It was a sensation that would last for hours after devouring a cheeseburger or the last slice of pepperoni pizza.

The final straw came during a business trip to Phoenix. I had yet another sinus infection. But this infection was a real killer. Along with the sinus pain and congestion, I was fatigued and had a raging fever that lasted the entire week. I could barely function. As I crawled into bed after another long day of meetings, I knew I couldn't go on like this. I needed to get to the bottom of whatever it was that was wrong with me and rule out any type of serious illness. The next morning, as the Arizona sun streamed into my hotel room, I placed a long distance call to my doctor and made an appointment.

∽

The Symptoms of Pancreatic Cancer

The symptoms of pancreatic cancer often don't appear until the disease is in an advanced stage. This makes early detection difficult. And, as you have seen from my experience, when symptoms do show up, they can be vague and nonspecific. Of course, this isn't exclusive to pancreatic cancer. Many types of cancer can sneak up on a patient because the symptoms can often be subtle. Symptoms can also vary depending on where the cancer is located and whether or not it has spread to other areas of the body. While not everyone experiences all of these signs, here are the most common symptoms of pancreatic cancer:

* **ABDOMINAL PAIN.** Usually in the upper abdomen. The pain may also radiate to the back and worsen when lying down or within a few hours of eating.

✳ **BLOATING.** Some people with pancreatic cancer feel full soon after they begin eating or experience uncomfortable swelling in the abdomen after a meal.

✳ **CHANGES IN STOOL AND URINE COLOR.** Urine may become quite dark, while stools lose their brown color, becoming a pale, clay color. This is often due to the bile duct being blocked. Stools can also have an odd, strong smell.

✳ **ELEVATED BLOOD SUGAR LEVELS.** Some people with pancreatic cancer unexpectedly develop diabetes as the cancer impairs the pancreas' ability to produce insulin. It is important to note, however, that most diabetes develops because of reasons unrelated to pancreatic cancer.

✳ **ITCHING.** Itchy skin is a less common symptom of pancreatic cancer. However, when coupled with abdominal pain or jaundice, it can be significant in making a more timely diagnosis. Unfortunately, when someone with undiagnosed pancreatic cancer is experiencing itchy skin, it is often misdiagnosed as a dermatological condition.

✳ **JAUNDICE.** A condition marked by the yellowing of the skin and eyes that commonly occurs in people with pancreatic cancer. This discoloration is due to an increased level of bilirubin—a yellow compound produced by the breakdown of hemoglobin from red blood cells. This buildup can occur when a tumor partially or completely blocks the bile ducts.

✳ **LOSS OF APPETITE.** Appetite loss is a symptom of hundreds of diseases and conditions, including pancreatic cancer. While this can be due to something as simple as a stomach virus, it can also signal something severe. When symptoms are vague like this, medical tests are necessary to make an accurate diagnosis.

✳ **NAUSEA AND/OR VOMITING.** Ignoring nonspecific symptoms, like nausea, often results in a delay in a pancreatic cancer diagnosis.

✳ **WEIGHT LOSS.** Losing weight without trying may be welcomed by many people, but it can also be a sign that something is wrong. While unintended weight loss is common in many conditions, including many types of cancer, it is usually one of the first symptoms experienced in pancreatic cancer, along with abdominal pain.

CHAPTER TWO

Testing 1, 2, 3

Mysteries are not necessarily miracles.
~ *Johann Wolfgang von Goethe*

As I sat in the waiting room of the doctor's office, my fingers flew across the keyboard of my laptop. *Why not get a little work done?*, I thought. But in the back of my mind, I wondered what was going on with my health and hoped the doctor could give me a quick fix for my ever-expanding problems. I just wanted to put my life back on track.

When I finally saw the doctor, I listed all of the problems I had been experiencing over the past few months—the colds, the sinus problems, the fatigue, the itching, and the constant indigestion. But instead of offering a magic solution to my symptoms, she decided to run a complete blood cell count and handed me a prescription for a proton pump inhibitor to help manage my digestive troubles. As the doctor turned and reached for the doorknob, I asked the question that had been nagging at the recesses of my mind for weeks. "I don't want to sound like I'm overreacting, but I thought you should know that my uncle recently passed away from pancreatic cancer. There's no way this could be that, right?" The doctor said that she would order a CT scan to rule it out.

My follow-up appointment allowed me to breathe a big sigh of relief. The blood work didn't raise any red flags. When I asked about the CT scan, the doctor smiled and said there was no evidence of any tumors. While I was thrilled at the news, I felt a little silly that I had pushed for the CT scan. CT scans are expensive, often costing thousands of dollars for a single test. But I wanted the peace of mind that it wasn't pancreatic or some other type of cancer.

Gathering Clues

Of course, even though the tests had ruled out cancer, the doctor still didn't have an answer as to what was causing my symptoms. But the signs seemed to point to my digestive tract. A visit to the gastroenterologist resulted in a recommendation for an endoscopic retrograde cholangiopancreatography (ERCP) to check the liver, gallbladder, bile ducts, and pancreas. ERCP is used primarily to diagnose and treat conditions of the bile ducts, including gallstones, inflammatory strictures (scars), leaks (from trauma and surgery), and cancer. It combines the use of X-rays and an endoscope, which is a long, flexible, lighted tube. Through the endoscope, the doctor can see the inside of the stomach and duodenum. This test also offers a glimpse—via X-ray—into the health of the bile ducts in the biliary tree and pancreas.

I checked into the University of Washington Medical Center on January 5, 2007. After donning a hospital gown, I met with Dr. Bruce Tung, the gastroenterologist who would be performing the test. He explained the procedure and said that he would remove any gallstones or "sludge" that may be blocking the bile duct. A blockage could very well be the cause of my jaundice and itchiness, as well as the pain I was feeling in my abdomen and back.

I was in good spirits as I was wheeled into the room where the procedure would take place. Maybe this would finally resolve my problems, I thought, as they administered a sedative to help me relax during the exam. Once the drugs kicked in, I barely realized that a tube was sliding down my throat. I would later learn that a scope was threaded through my esophagus, stomach, and duodenum until it reached the spot where the ducts of the biliary tree and pancreas open into the duodenum. I don't remember being turned onto my stomach as the doctor inserted a small plastic tube through the scope. Through the tube, the physician injected dye into the ducts to make them show up clearly on the X-rays.

Once the test was over, the doctor told Gwen and me that he had, indeed, found and cleared a blockage. He also performed a sphincterotomy to widen the opening of the bile duct. With any luck, this would ensure that any future stones or sludge could easily pass. As Gwen drove me home, I looked forward to getting a good night's sleep and then resuming my life. No such luck. Two days later I was in the emergency room suffering from a rare bout of internal bleeding from the sphincterotomy. Fortunately, it wasn't a critical complication, and the bleeding eventually stopped on its own. But it was a strong indication that my ordeal was far from over.

Indeed, during a follow-up appointment the day before Valentine's Day, I was diagnosed with an inflamed pancreas, a condition called pancreatitis. That could explain the bloating, back and abdominal pain, muscles aches, and dark urine. Of more concern, my enzyme levels were off the charts. My liver enzymes, which should be between 38 and 110, had soared to 694. My digestive enzymes weren't any better. Amylase, an enzyme produced in the pancreas and salivary glands that helps digest starches, was more than twice the normal levels. And my levels of lipase—an enzyme secreted in the digestive tract that breaks down fats—were a whopping 276. Normal levels are below 30.

Instead of surprising Gwen with candy and flowers, this Valentine's Day would bring the stark realization for both of us that something was terribly wrong. The next week, I found myself in the hospital for a second ERCP. While my symptoms were much the same as I had experienced before the first ERCP, this time there weren't any gallstones or sludge. But the area around the sphincterotomy was extremely swollen and would bleed at the slightest irritation. This wasn't surprising since pancreatitis can cause swelling that blocks the bile duct. The gastroenterologist who performed the second ERCP put in a temporary stent to hold the bile duct open.

Good News, Bad News

Along with all this poking and prodding inside my digestive tract was a battery of other tests, including additional CT scans. The results from the most recent scan, however, offered another ray of hope—there was still no evidence of cancer or any cysts on my pancreas.

That welcome news was tempered with the fact that my enzyme levels were still terribly out of whack. While my liver enzymes were a bit lower, my amylase and lipase levels had skyrocketed. Everyone was stumped. The stent should have helped to regulate my enzyme levels. Instead, they had gone from bad to worse.

Finding Answers

COMMON DIAGNOSTIC TESTS

Diagnosing pancreatic cancer often doesn't occur until a patient has been suffering from symptoms for weeks or months. Since many of the symptoms can point to other problems besides pancreatic cancer, a doctor will typically begin to search for the cause using a battery of tests. Below are the most typical tests that doctors can choose from to confirm or rule out the disease.

* **HISTORY AND PHYSICAL EXAM.** The first step is to determine if you have any risk factors for pancreatic cancer. This is done by compiling a complete medical history and documenting information about the symptoms you are experiencing. A thorough physical exam will be conducted with a focus on the abdomen to check for any masses or fluid buildup. The skin and the white part of the eyes will be checked for jaundice. Cancers that block the bile duct may also cause the gallbladder to become enlarged. This can sometimes be felt during a physical exam. If the doctor strongly suspects pancreatic cancer, he may check other areas of the body—especially the liver and lymph nodes—to see if there is any evidence that the cancer has spread.

* **BLOOD TESTS.** Several types of blood tests can be used to help diagnose pancreatic cancer or to help determine treatment options if it is found. Blood tests that measure bilirubin (a chemical made by the liver) can help determine if jaundice is due to liver disease or blocked bile flow. Elevated blood levels of the tumor markers CA 19-9 and carcinoembryonic antigen (CEA) may point to pancreatic cancer, but these tests aren't always accurate.

  Other blood tests that evaluate certain pancreatic hormones can help diagnose specific kinds of tumors such as pancreatic neuroendocrine tumors that interact with both the body's hormonal system and the nervous system or tumors that produce insulin. These tests measure insulin, glucose, and a byproduct of insulin production called C-peptide, as well as other pancreatic hormones like gastrin, glucagon, somatostatin, pancreatic polypeptide, and vasoactive intestinal peptide. Together these tests can help diagnose pancreatic cancer.

  Currently, one biopharmaceutical company is looking into a new type of blood test that may be able to detect pancreatic cancer in its early stages, when it's most curable. The test uses an antibody that works like a heat-seeking missile, homing in on and attaching to cells that carry a protein called PAM4 that is present in the vast majority of pancreatic cancers. The antibody also shows promise for treating the disease by acting as a carrier for radiation or drugs that can target and kill pancreatic cancer cells.

Researchers first tried the test on blood samples taken from nearly 300 people. Some of the participants had pancreatic cancer, but others were either healthy or had been diagnosed with other types of cancer, including breast and lung cancer. The test was positive in 77 percent of pancreatic patients, but only in 5 percent of patients with other forms of cancer. A second study evaluated the PAM4 protein test in 68 people who had had pancreatic cancer surgery, as well as 19 healthy people. The test correctly detected 62 percent of very early-stage pancreatic cancers that were still confined to the pancreas, 86 percent of cases that had spread to nearby tissue, and 91 percent of late-stage cancers that had spread to distant sites in the body. Overall, the test correctly identified 81 percent of all pancreatic cancers.

While it may take two or three years before this test is available, it could prove to be a lifesaving tool for anyone at risk of pancreatic cancer. In my opinion, it can't come soon enough.

❋ **Computed Tomography (CT, CAT) Scan.** This is an X-ray that provides detailed cross-sectional images of your body. Instead of taking one picture, like a standard X-ray, a CT scanner takes many pictures as it rotates around you. A computer then combines these pictures into images that resemble slices of the part of your body being studied.

Before your scan, you may be asked to drink a liquid called oral contrast. This helps outline the intestine so certain areas are not mistaken for tumors. You may also receive an intravenous line through which a different kind of contrast dye (IV contrast) is injected. This helps better outline structures in your body. During the test—which is painless—you will lie on a table that moves in and out of a doughnut-shaped scanner. These scans show the pancreas fairly clearly and often can confirm the location of the cancer. CT scans can also show the organs near the pancreas, as well as lymph nodes and distant organs to where the cancer might have spread. The CT scan can also help to determine whether surgery is a good treatment option. However, while a CT scan is a very sound diagnostic technique in many situations, in my case it did not reveal my cancer. Instead, it was discovered a month later during a PET-CT scan. This scan not only identified the cancer, it also showed just how far it had spread.

* **MAGNETIC RESONANCE IMAGING (MRI).** This imaging test uses radio waves and strong magnets instead of X-rays. The energy from the radio waves is absorbed by the body and then released in a pattern formed by the type of body tissue scanned and by certain diseases. A computer translates the pattern into a detailed image. Not only does this produce cross-sectional slices of the body like a CT scanner, it also produces slices that are parallel with the length of the body. A contrast material might be injected just as with CT scans, this but this is used less often. Most doctors prefer CT scans to look at the pancreas, but an MRI can sometimes provide additional information.

  MRI scans are more uncomfortable than CT scans, and they can take up to an hour to complete. Typically, you will lie inside a narrow tube, which can feel confining. However, newer "open-sided" MRI machines can reduce claustrophobic feelings. Since the MRI machine is loud, some testing facilities provide headphones with music to block out the noise.

* **SOMATOSTATIN RECEPTOR SCINTIGRAPHY.** Also called an OctreoScan, this test can be very helpful in the diagnosis of pancreatic neuroendocrine tumors. It uses a hormone-like substance called octreotide that has been bound to radioactive indium-111, an isotope that emits radioactivity as it disintegrates. A small amount of this substance is injected into a vein; it travels through the bloodstream and is attracted to neuroendocrine tumors. About four hours after the injection, a special camera can be used to show where the radioactivity has collected in the body. Additional scans may be done on the following days as well.

* **POSITRON EMISSION TOMOGRAPHY (PET) SCAN.** PET scans begin with the injection of glucose that contains a radioactive atom into the blood. Because cancer cells grow rapidly, they absorb more of the radioactive sugar than normal cells do. A special camera then creates a picture that highlights these areas of radioactivity. The

picture is not finely detailed like a CT or MRI scan, but it provides helpful information, especially if the cancer has spread.

* **ULTRASOUND.** This technology uses sound waves to produce images of internal organs like the pancreas. For an abdominal ultrasound, a wand-shaped probe called a transducer is placed on the skin of the abdomen. It emits sound waves and detects the echoes as they bounce off internal organs. The pattern of echoes is processed by a computer to produce an image on a screen. The echoes made by most pancreatic tumors differ from those of normal pancreatic tissue.

  Endoscopic ultrasound is more accurate than an abdominal ultrasound. This test is done with an ultrasound probe that is attached to an endoscope. You will be sedated before the probe is passed through the mouth or nose to the esophagus, stomach, and the first part of the small intestine. The probe can then be pointed toward the pancreas, which sits next to the small intestine. The probe is on the tip of the endoscope, so it can get very close to the area where the tumor is to take pictures. This is a very good way to look at the pancreas. It is better than CT scans for spotting small tumors. If a tumor is found, a biopsy can then be performed.

* **ENDOSCOPIC RETROGRADE CHOLANGIOPANCREATOGRAPHY (ERCP).** As you learned from my experience, ERCP is performed by passing an endoscope down the throat until it makes its way into the first part of the small intestine. The doctor can see through the endoscope to find the ampulla of Vater (the place where the common bile duct is connected to the small intestine). A small amount of dye is then injected through the tube into the common bile duct and X-rays are taken. This dye helps outline the bile duct and pancreatic duct. The X-ray can show narrowing or blockage of these ducts that might be due to pancreatic cancer. The doctor doing this test can also put a small brush through the tube to remove cells for a biopsy. This procedure is usually done while the patient is sedated. As occurred during my second ERCP, a stent can be placed in the bile duct to keep it open if necessary.

* **ANGIOGRAPHY.** This is an X-ray procedure that looks at blood flow. A small amount of contrast dye is injected into an artery to outline the blood vessels. After this, X-rays are taken to determine whether blood flow in a particular area is blocked or compressed by a tumor.

❧

It can also show any abnormal blood vessels in the area. This test can be useful in finding out if a pancreatic cancer has grown through the walls of certain blood vessels. Mainly, it helps surgeons decide whether the cancer can be completely removed without damaging vital blood vessels. Angiography can also be used to look for pancreatic neuroendocrine tumors that are too small to be seen on other imaging tests. These tumors cause the body to make extra blood vessels that "feed" the tumor, and these surplus blood vessels can be seen on angiography.

Angiography can be uncomfortable because a small catheter must be placed into the artery leading to the pancreas. Usually the catheter is put into an artery in your inner thigh and threaded up to the pancreas. A local anesthetic is often used to numb the area before inserting the catheter. Then the dye is injected quickly to outline all the blood vessels while the X-rays are being taken.

✱ **BIOPSY.** While all of these tests can point to pancreatic cancer, the only way to know whether a tumor is cancerous is to remove a small piece of and look at it under the microscope. There are several types of biopsies. The procedure used most often to diagnose pancreatic cancer is called a fine needle aspiration (FNA) biopsy. For this test, a doctor inserts a thin needle through the skin and into the pancreas. The doctor uses CT scan images or endoscopic ultrasonography to view the position of the needle and make sure that it is in the tumor. Doctors can also biopsy the tumor by using the endoscopic

One thing that everyone agreed on was that I was suffering from severe pancreatitis and gall bladder issues. The solution? Remove the gall bladder. But first, Dr. Tung decided to have another gastroenterologist—Dr. Michael Saunders—perform one last test, an endoscopic ultrasound and a biopsy of the inflamed ampullary tissue.

March 23, 2007. I was in my home office when Dr. Saunders called and delivered the news. Luckily, I was sitting down. For months, my constellation of symptoms—the fatigue, infections, jaundice, and elevated pancreatic enzyme levels—had puzzled my gastroenterologists. But the mystery was finally solved. Dr. Saunders explained that the biopsy taken from my ampulla confirmed the presence of cancer. There was a high probability that the cancer was not confined to the ampulla. My

ultrasound to place the needle directly through the wall of the duo-denum into the tumor. In either case, small tissue samples can be removed through the needle.

In the past, surgical biopsies, in which an incision is made through the skin into the wall of the abdomen to examine internal organs, were common. Surgical biopsies allow a surgeon to use a scalpel or a needle to remove a small portion of tissue in areas that look or feel abnormal. Although surgical biopsies once required a large incision—with general anesthesia and a hospital stay—less inva-sive procedures are now available. Using laparoscopy, the surgeon makes several small incisions and inserts small telescope-like instru-ments into the abdominal cavity. One of these is usually connected to a video monitor. The surgeon can view the abdomen and see how big the tumor is and whether it has spread. He may take tissue samples as well.

Most doctors who treat pancreatic cancer try to avoid surgery unless imaging tests suggest that an operation might be able to remove all of the visible cancer. Even after doing imaging tests and laparoscopy, there are times when the surgeon begins an operation with the intent of removing the cancer but finds dur-ing surgery that it has spread too far to be removed completely. In these cases, a sample of the cancer is taken only to confirm the diagnosis, and the rest of the planned operation is stopped.

Source: American Cancer Society

pancreas could also be involved. Subsequent surgery would later dis-cover that cancer riddled my pancreas, bilary tract, small bowel, and colon. At the time, the surgeon postulated that the cancer originated from my pancreas, although subsequent biopsy analysis cast some doubt about my cancer's true origin.

Pancreatic Cancer

With all of this talk about pancreatic cancer, I suppose I should spend a few minutes explaining a bit about the pancreas itself. The pancreas is about six inches long and looks sort of like a pear lying on its side. But even though it may be small, it is a crucial part of the digestive system. This vital organ secretes hormones, including insulin and glucagons. These two hormones are especially important for the maintenance of blood sugar, since insulin lowers blood sugar levels and glucagon increases them according to what the body needs at any particular moment. The pancreas also produces digestive enzymes like amylase, which digests starch; lipase, which breaks down fats; and trypsin, a protein processor.

The pancreas is covered with a thin connective tissue that divides it into lobes. The head, which is the right section of the pancreas, is the largest portion and lies in the first curve of the small intestine. The smallest part of the pancreas is the tail, which ends near the spleen.

The pancreas also contains two different types of tissue: groups of cells called the islets of Langerhans, and ducts called the pancreatic acini. The islets of Langerhans, which is also known as the endocrine pancreas, is the portion of the pancreas that manufactures and secretes hormones. The pancreatic acini, also called the exocrine pancreas, makes and secretes pancreatic enzymes, as well as bicarbonate that is used to neutralize stomach acids.

Pancreatic cancer develops when cells in the pancreas don't die when they should—a process called apoptosis. Cells throughout the body are normally programmed to die in a controlled way that regulates and maintains the proper number of cells in various tissues. This process is sometimes referred to as cellular suicide. One reason this happens is to get rid of damaged cells that could be harmful to the rest of the organism, such as ones that will eventually become cancerous. Apoptosis, or the lack thereof, is a key factor in whether or not cancer will develop.

About 95 percent of pancreatic cancers begin in the exocrine pancreas, where enzymes are produced. The remaining 5 percent are cancers of the endocrine pancreas, where hormones are produced. These are also called islet cell cancers.

Many factors can trigger the growth of cancer cells in the pancreas, which I'll talk about in the next chapter. But the thing about this type of cancer cell is that it's sneaky. Unlike some types of tumor cells that can be easily detected, pancreatic cancer cells escape detection by hiding out in the recesses of the pancreas. Even after they are detected, they may seem to come and go. And when they reappear, they can grow aggressively. Typically, pancreatic cancer spreads first to nearby lymph nodes, then to the liver. In some cases, it can also travel to the lungs. What's more, it can invade the surrounding organs like the upper region of the small intestine, the stomach, and the colon.

A SPOUSE'S PERSPECTIVE: Hearing the News

"Go ahead."

Those two words from Mark were all I needed to hear to start the ball rolling on our long-awaited kitchen remodel. After years of waiting and wishing, I finally placed the order for new cabinets and told our kitchen designer which countertop we wanted. At that moment, the most pressing concern in my mind was deciding which sink and faucet to order. Excitement was in the air.

Over the years, windows, doors, a furnace, a water heater, and a roof have been replaced in this house. Ho hum. But remodeling a room—especially a kitchen—was life-changing, and I couldn't wait to share the kitchen transformation with Mark. As I skipped into Mark's home office, he was just finishing up a phone call from Dr. Saunders. I stopped in my tracks. To this very day, the devastated yet stoic expression on Mark's face is painfully etched into my memory. It was a horrified and stunned look I wish to forever forget.

"Gwen, it's not good. I have cancer."

Mark held me a long, long time as my tears flowed. I was shocked, confused, and very afraid.

"How could you have cancer when so many tests were negative?"

"I've never heard of the ampulla. What is it?"

"If only it was your gall bladder."

"How do we tell the boys?"

Mark insisted that we keep the new cabinets I had ordered, but any thoughts of a new kitchen became unbearable. A day that had begun with such high hopes ended with our family's worst nightmare.

— *Gwen*

Pancreatic cancer starts to wreak havoc long before symptoms appear by changing the way the pancreas works. It can create an imbalance of pancreatic enzymes, bicarbonate, and bile salt. It also impairs how the body uses these pancreatic enzymes. What's more, pancreatic cancer causes poor nutrient absorption from the foods you eat. This can prevent potentially beneficial nutrients from being utilized to slow the growth of the cancer.

Setting the Stage

Dr. Saunders explained that pancreatic cancer had been confirmed from a tissue sample from my ampulla. The fact that the cancer had occurred relatively early in life—I was just 47 years old—was worrisome. When

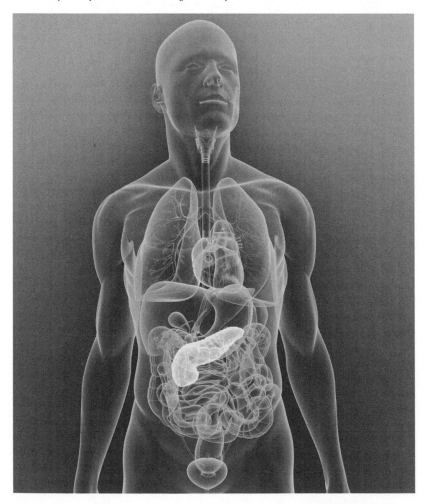

cancer appears at such a relatively early age, it can be indicative of an aggressive cancer. And so it was. Another PET-CT scan showed that my cancer was on the move. It was using my lymphatic system like an interstate highway to spread to my neck, chest, and abdomen.

Indications from a future surgery suggested that the cancer was stage 4 pancreatic cancer. This would be the worst possible news I could get.

When it comes to cancer, staging describes whether the cancer has spread and, if so, what parts of the body are affected. This is important because treatment is often decided according to the stage of a cancer. Many of the same tests the doctor uses to diagnose pancreatic cancer can also help determine the stage of the disease.

According to the National Cancer Institute, there are three ways that cancer can spread in the body. First, cancer cells can invade the surrounding normal tissue. It can also travel through the lymph system to

THE STAGES OF PANCREATIC CANCER		
Stage	**Description**	**% of Cases**
0	Abnormal cells are found in the lining of the pancreas. Also called carcinoma in situ.	N/A
IA	Cancer has formed but is limited to the pancreas. The tumor is 2 cm or smaller.	<5
IB	Same as 1A, but the tumor is larger than 2 cm.	
IIA	Cancer has spread to nearby organs like the duodenum or bile duct but has not entered the lymph nodes. This means that although the cancer has been growing locally, there is a chance that it may not have spread through the blood or lymph systems.	10
IIB	Cancer may have grown into the tissues surrounding the pancreas and may have spread to the nearby lymph nodes.	
III	Cancer is growing outside the pancreas into nearby organs such as the stomach, spleen, and colon, and to nearby large blood vessels or major nerves. It may or may not have spread into nearby lymph nodes.	30
IV	Cancer has spread to distant organs like the liver, lung, and peritoneal cavity.	60

other places in the body. Finally, cancer can spread through the blood. When this occurs, the cancer invades the veins and capillaries and travels to other organs and structures in the body.

When cancer cells break away from the primary tumor and travel through the lymph or blood to other locations, a secondary tumor may form. This process is known as metastasis. The secondary tumor is the same type of cancer as the primary tumor. In other words, if pancreatic cancer spreads to the lung, the cancer cells in the lung are actually pancreatic cancer cells. The disease is metastatic pancreatic cancer, not lung cancer.

TNM Stages of Pancreatic Cancer

TNM stands for *tumor, node,* and *metastasis.* This system describes the size of a primary tumor (T), whether there are lymph nodes with cancer cells in them (N), and if the cancer has spread to a different body parts (M).

* **T STAGES.** There are five stages of tumor size in pancreatic cancer. T (carcinoma in situ) is the smallest and T4 is the largest.

* **N STAGES.** There are two main N stages. They indicate whether the pancreatic cancer has spread to the lymph nodes (N1) or not (N0).

* **M STAGES.** There are two M stages to indicate whether the cancer has spread to distant body parts, like the liver or lungs (M1) or not (M0).

Most doctors and researchers measure tumors in centimeters. This can be hard for patients to visualize. In the diagram below, a pea, peanut, walnut, and lime represent tumor sizes.

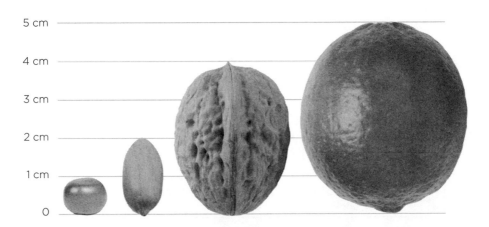

CHAPTER THREE

How Did This Happen?

Being sorry for myself is a luxury
I can't afford.
~ *Stephen King*

PANCREATIC CANCER IS THE DEADLIEST TYPE of cancer there is. Because it is very aggressive and typically not discovered until it's in an advanced stage, the survival rate is the worst of any cancer. Eighty percent of people diagnosed with the disease can only expect to live another five to eight months.

I'm in real trouble.

A million thoughts popped into my head the minute I heard my diagnosis. I thought of my family. How I had looked forward to watching my sons grow up, get married, and have children of their own. It was a future that appeared to vanish with those four little words: *You have pancreatic cancer.* In all likelihood, there would be no time for leisurely advice from their father. No growing old with Gwen. No time . . .

I'm not ready to check out yet. There are simply too many things I have left to do.

Anytime someone is diagnosed with a potentially fatal disease, they are overwhelmed with thoughts and emotion. Some people are paralyzed with fear, some with sadness. Anxiety, helplessness, anger, and even defiance are common. Everyone is different and so everyone experiences this kind of life-changing news differently. But, after the initial shock wears off, most people—myself included—start to wonder why this hideous disease has taken up residence inside their body. Was it something I did? Was I exposed to something that triggered the cancerous mutations?

I grew up in a major city and was exposed to all of the nasty pollutants that millions of other city-dwellers are exposed to each and every year. But there's nothing that jumps out as a red flag. Our house wasn't situated under power lines or built over a Superfund site. The only thing that even remotely stands out was the summer job I once had with an electronics manufacturer. I would spend my days calibrating the liquid flow of the devices they made, never questioning the health impact of having my hands bathed in noxious-smelling chemicals day in and day out.

Heredity could have played a role. There is a history of gastrointestinal cancer on both sides of my family tree. Liver and stomach cancer are common among Asian Americans, and my family was no exception. Both my father's father and my mother's mother passed away from

How deadly is pancreatic cancer? In 2009 alone, 42,470 people were diagnosed with the disease. Of those, about 35,240 people died within a year of diagnosis. Overall, only 20 percent of people with pancreatic cancer live at least one year after diagnosis, and less than 4 percent will be alive after 5 years. The following charts put these statistics into sobering perspective.

5-YEAR SURVIVAL RATE FOR EXOCRINE PANCREATIC CANCER

Stage IA	37%
Stage IB	21%
Stage IIA	12%
Stage IIB	6%
Stage III	2%
Stage IV	1%

5-YEAR SURVIVAL RATE FOR PANCREATIC NEUROENDOCRINE TUMORS

Localized	87%
Regional	70%
Distant	24%

gastrointestinal cancer. And then there was my Uncle Nobi, who died of pancreatic cancer just months before my own diagnosis. But this may not have as much to do with being of Japanese heritage as the lifestyle my ancestors adopted once they arrived in America. Epidemiological studies show that Asians who adopt the eating habits of their new country—the standard American diet based largely on heavy meat, fat, and sugar consumption—experience a sharp increase in their risk of developing gastrointestinal cancer.

I know that I have embraced the standard American diet (with the ironic acronym SAD) with gusto for most of my life. During my college days, I devoured at least one cheeseburger every day. After graduation, I traded in my beloved burgers for pizza—and not just any pizza. Required toppings included double cheese, pepperoni, sausage, ham, bacon, and beef. It's no exaggeration to say that our neighborhood pizza delivery was on speed-dial and my freezer was well-stocked with frozen pepperoni pies.

Going out to eat meant fried fish, fried chicken, and, of course, French fries. I kept eating this way even as I got older and my cholesterol levels edged into dangerous territory. As a pharmacist, I knew that cholesterol-lowering statin drugs could help prevent a heart attack in spite of my diet. So I popped my daily Lipitor and ate whatever I wanted, never giving a second thought to what my diet was doing to my gastrointestinal tract.

While I overindulged in unhealthy food, I shortchanged myself in the sleep department. As a workaholic with many commitments, I would work a full day, come home and spend a few hours with the family, then steal off to my home office to burn the midnight oil armed, of course, with my late-night pepperoni pizza. Sleep was a luxury, and I averaged a mere four hours per night for many years. It was enough, or so I thought. What I've come to realize since my diagnosis, however, is that sleep is vital to a healthy immune system. Had I allowed myself more time to rest, my body may have had a better chance at fighting off rogue cancer cells.

But I felt invincible. I had plenty of energy and rarely, if ever, got sick. I thought I could keep this up forever. I was wrong. For those readers in denial about their own unwholesome habits, I am living proof that an unhealthy life eventually catches up with you

Risky Business

It's not surprising that the same factors come into play whether you are trying to pinpoint the cause of your cancer or looking for ways to prevent the disease. Some of the risk factors linked to pancreatic cancer are things you can't do anything about. But, as you will see, many are well within your control.

RISK FACTORS THAT CANNOT BE MODIFIED

AGE. The risk of developing pancreatic cancer goes up as you get older. Almost all pancreatic cancer patients have passed their 45th birthday. Nearly 90 percent are older than 55 years, and more than 70 percent are 65 years old or older. While the average age at the time of diagnosis is 72, don't make the mistake of thinking this is a disease reserved for the elderly. Patrick Swayze was 56 when diagnosed. Michael Landon was 54. Playwright Lorraine Hansberry (*Raisin in the Sun*) was 34, and comedian Bill Hicks was 32. As for me? While not famous, I was just 47 when I was diagnosed.

DIABETES. Exocrine pancreatic cancer is more common in people with type 2 diabetes, but it's hard to tell if diabetes increases the risk of pancreatic cancer or if the cancer triggers the diabetes by reducing the amount of insulin produced by the pancreas. An Australian study of more than 9,200 people with pancreatic cancer found that, while long-standing diabetes may increase risk slightly, new-onset diabetes is more likely to signal the presence of underlying cancer. Complicating the issue further are recent studies suggesting that certain treatments for diabetes may either decrease or increase the risk of pancreatic cancer.

ETHNICITY. While no one knows why, African Americans are at higher risk of pancreatic cancer than either Caucasians or Asians—and Caucasians have a slightly higher risk than those of Asian descent.

FAMILY HISTORY AND GENETICS. Cancer, including pancreatic cancer, can run in families. There are a couple of reasons for this phenomenon. Since cracking the genetic code, researchers have begun looking at certain genetic mutations that can be inherited. Inherited gene mutations are abnormal copies of certain genes that can be passed from parent to child. Two genetic mutations that are causing a lot of buzz in scientific circles are mutations in the cationic trypsinogen gene known as PRSS1 and mutations in a gene known as Von Hippel-Lindau (VHL) that can lead to an increased risk of pancreatic cancer and carcinoma of the ampulla of Vater.

Pancreatic neuroendocrine tumors and cancers can also be caused by a genetic syndrome. For instance, neurofibromatosis type 1 is caused by mutations in the gene NF1. This syndrome leads to an increased risk of tumors in the pancreas and interferes with somatostatin, a pancreatic hormone that controls the rate of nutrient absorption along with the release of insulin, glucagons, and other digestive hormones. Multiple endocrine neoplasia, type 1, caused by mutations in the gene MEN1, also leads to an increased risk of tumors of the islet cells of the pancreas, as well as in the parathyroid and pituitary glands.

But, being genetically predisposed to pancreatic cancer doesn't necessarily mean it's your destiny. Learned behavior—whether or not you have been raised to eat a healthful diet, stay active, and avoid bad habits like smoking—can play a much larger role in determining your risk of developing the disease, whether or not you carry the genes I've discussed. According to the new field of epigenetics, behavior and environment may be able to turn the table on faulty genes by changing the way they express themselves. In other words, nurture may be able to trump nature. If you are genetically predisposed toward pancreatic cancer or other life-threatening diseases, it's critical to be diligent about maintaining a healthy diet and lifestyle. You just might have more control than you think.

GENDER. Pancreatic cancer is an equal opportunity disease, but men have always been slightly more likely to develop this type of cancer largely because they were more likely to smoke. However, that gap is closing as more women now smoke.

HELICOBACTER PYLORI (*H. PYLORI*). The bacteria that cause ulcers may increase the odds of developing pancreatic cancer. Some researchers believe that excess stomach acid may also increase risk.

CHRONIC PANCREATITIS. This long-term infection of the pancreas is linked to an increased risk of pancreatic cancer. This link is strongest in smokers; however, a small number of cases appear to be caused by an inherited gene mutation that can boost the odds of developing pancreatic cancer by up to 74 percent.

RISK FACTORS YOU CAN CHANGE

ALCOHOL USE. Drinking on a daily basis modestly increases pancreatic cancer risk. According to a recent review that looked at 14 studies, the risk of developing pancreatic cancer was 22 percent higher in people who had two or more drinks daily compared to teetotalers. The risk was highest among those who drank mixed drinks like margaritas or martinis, but overindulging in beer and wine also increased risk.

COFFEE CONSUMPTION. Some studies have suggested that drinking coffee increases the risk of pancreatic cancer via a mutation of the KRAS gene. The KRAS gene acts like a molecular on/off switch that, when turned on, recruits and activates proteins necessary for the propagation of growth factor. But when a mutation occurs, the KRAS gene can turn a normal cell into a tumor cell. What causes the KRAS gene to go rogue? Some scientists speculate that it could be the organochlorine pesticides used to grow coffee. Since I don't indulge in either alcohol or coffee, this wasn't an issue for me. But, if you can't survive without your morning cuppa Joe, it might be smart to switch to an organically grown brand.

DIET. As I hinted at earlier, what you eat can raise your risk of pancreatic cancer. The U.S. National Cancer Institute recently published a report that links a diet high in animal fats to pancreatic cancer. The Cancer Institute's research team gathered data from more than half a million people in 1995 and 1996. Of those, 1,337 people developed pancreatic cancer. It turns out that the men who ate diets high in animal fats had a 53 percent higher risk for developing pancreatic cancer than those who ate the least amount of animal fats. Women eating a lot of animal fat had a 23 percent increased risk. All meat—especially beef, pork, and processed meat (sausage, bacon, and lunch meat)—is high in animal fat. Full-fat cheese and full-fat dairy products also pack a high saturated fat punch.

Recent research from Sweden found that sugar intake is also strongly linked to pancreatic cancer. The seven-year study involved 77,797 healthy men and women over the age of 45. None of the participants had a history of either cancer or diabetes. The researchers looked at the amount of sugar the participants ate and pinpointed three main sugar sources that were strong predictors of pancreatic cancer:

* High added sugar intake (sugar added to coffee, tea, cereal, etc.) was associated with a 69 percent higher risk of developing pancreatic cancer than a low sugar intake.

* Drinking two or more soft drinks daily was associated with a 93 percent greater chance of getting pancreatic cancer than low soft drink consumption.

* A high intake of sugar-sweetened fruit increased pancreatic cancer risk by 51 percent.

But refined sugar isn't the only type of carbohydrate you need to worry about. A diet high in simple carbohydrates like refined pasta, white bread, white rice, cookies, and crackers, can raise your blood sugar levels. This can boost your risk of pancreatic cancer, too. During one 10-year study, investigators examined data from the Korean Cancer Prevention Study, which involved more than 1.2 million Koreans between the ages of 30 and 95. They found that pancreatic cancer was strongly associated with blood sugar levels. Women with the highest blood sugar levels had more than twice the risk of pancreatic cancer compared to those in the lowest group while men in the highest group had a 91 percent increased risk of pancreatic cancer.

LACK OF EXERCISE. While a sedentary lifestyle won't automatically set you up for pancreatic or other types of cancer, a lack of physical activity contributes to other risk factors like obesity. What's more, people who don't exercise on a regular basis are more likely to have unhealthy eating habits that can make them vulnerable. On the flip side, studies show that exercise has a protective effect against a slew of diseases, including pancreatic cancer.

OBESITY. People who are obese are 72 percent more likely to be diagnosed with pancreatic cancer compared to those who aren't obese or overweight. And women who have central or abdominal obesity—especially if they are postmenopausal—have a 70 percent higher risk of the disease than their slim counterparts. Researchers believe that obesity increases the risk of pancreatic cancer by affecting insulin levels. Being overweight may also amplify the effect of alcohol consumption and smoking on pancreatic cancer.

Obesity also greatly increases the chance that cancer will spread to other parts of the body. According to a study of pancreatic cancer patients conducted at the University of Texas M. D. Anderson Cancer Center, those with a body mass index (BMI) of more than 35 kg/m² had a 12-fold higher risk for lymph node metastases and almost twice the risk for cancer recurrence and death compared with normal-weight patients.

When I was diagnosed, I had a BMI of 28—not obese by any means, but enough to peg me as overweight. This, combined with my other risk factors, may have pushed me over the pancreatic cancer precipice.

OCCUPATIONAL EXPOSURE. Exposure to certain chemicals in the workplace can contribute to the development of pancreatic cancer. Not surprisingly, industries associated with a heightened risk include printing and paper manufacturing, chemical or petroleum processing, and medical testing. Farm workers who are routinely exposed to pesticides also have a greater chance of developing pancreatic cancer.

Which compounds are linked to the highest risk? According to researchers in Finland, petroleum-based chlorinated hydrocarbons used to make tires, tennis shoes, anesthetics, industrial solvents, and pesticides pose the most risk. Job-related exposure to nickel and chromium can also increase your odds. Other workplace threats include polycyclic aromatic hydrocarbons (PAHs), organochlorine insecticides, silica dust, and aliphatic and alicyclic hydrocarbon solvents used in printing.

SMOKING. The risk of developing pancreatic cancer is two to three times higher if you smoke. Researchers at Michigan State University recently found that PAHs—the chemicals produced by burning tobacco products—interfere with the communication between the body's cells. More importantly, the study showed that some of these chemicals don't necessarily initiate the cancer, but rather contribute to its progression. But it isn't just the smoke. People who use smokeless tobacco also have a higher risk of pancreatic cancer. New evidence from Columbia University in New York shows that smokeless tobacco changes the shape of pancreatic cells and prevents the pancreas from functioning normally. And both cigarette smoke and smokeless tobacco trigger chronic inflammation that creates oxidative stress and damages the DNA in cells.

About 20 to 30 percent of exocrine pancreatic cancer cases are thought to be caused by cigarette smoking. Many experts think that smoking explains why the rate of pancreatic cancer had been increasing in the last 50 years and is only now starting to decline as smoking rates have dropped.

This may seem like an overwhelming list, but tackling just one or two of the modifiable risk factors can improve your odds of maintaining good health. Had someone given me a rundown of the many ways I was jeopardizing my health with my bad habits, perhaps I might have changed my ways. At least I like to think so. Instead, I can only share what I've learned in the hopes that it may save someone else.

Pity Is a Four-Letter Word

It's natural to try and figure out why something happens. But, when it comes to cancer, it usually occurs due to a combination of factors over a lifetime, making it all but impossible to target the exposure or activity that triggered its development. It's a futile exercise once you've been diagnosed with pancreatic cancer. What's done is done and you can't change the past.

I've seen many people with a terminal illness succumb to depression and self-pity once they learn of their fate. They give up, withdraw, and let the disease take its course. But that's not the route I choose to take. I may wonder what led to my disease, but I refuse to feel depressed, angry, or sorry for myself. I will not give cancer that much power over me and I will not allow it to define me.

Had I known that I had some of the risk factors for pancreatic cancer, maybe I would have done things differently. Maybe the cancer could have been detected at an earlier stage. But maybe doesn't change the reality. Instead I focus on the future and on the positive things I can do with the life I have left.

Maybe I can help someone else facing a devastating disease or life-changing crisis. Maybe I can educate others so that they can avoid my fate. Maybe this cancer that is eating away at me can be used to help others in ways I can't even fathom. A "gift" from God, if you will, that gives me purpose.

Gwen once said, "Wouldn't it be great if you could change history and avoid cancer and all of the suffering it brings?" At first, I thought it would indeed be wonderful. But, after a few minutes I realized that I wouldn't change a thing. Now, I know that this might sound crazy to most people. Nobody would actively choose cancer. No. If this had not landed on my plate, I certainly wouldn't have chosen it. Cancer can, however, be transformative. It's true that pancreatic cancer may shorten the duration of my life, but it has intensified the quality. Everything takes on a sense of urgency—tomorrow's goals need to get today's attention.

If you knew the Earth would be destroyed on a specific date, how would it change your life? Your priorities would no doubt change. Your relationship to those you love would take on a deeper, more immediate focus. Perhaps you would try to do all of the things that were important to you. The same thing happens when you are diagnosed with terminal cancer. You realize that you don't have all the time in the world. It's a lesson we would all do well to learn. You never know what the future holds—don't wait for something to rock your world before making positive changes. Making those changes now will enrich your life in ways you can't possibly imagine.

Cancer gave my life perspective. Trivial pursuits and meaningless activities have fallen by the wayside. Family and faith were always at the center of my existence. Now, both have taken on a much deeper meaning. From a practical standpoint, I have made it a priority to provide for my family financially. But dollars can be replaced. Memories can't. So I spend as much time as possible building memories for my two sons, James, 20, and Lane, 17—enough, I hope, to last a lifetime. Gwen and I savor our time together.

Through everything, my faith sustains me. A key part of my cancer recovery is a devout faith in God and belief He has a path for me to follow. Too often, people search for answers outside of themselves. Yet I truly believe that what they are looking for can be found within. In the final analysis, faith comes from inside and a person with faith can find his way, no matter what life throws at him.

I have also learned the importance of living in the moment. When you exist only in the present, you engage yourself completely. The future doesn't exist and the past does not hold you back. Living in the moment is about just being. If you are fully present in every situation, you experience everything totally and absolutely. Even everyday activities warrant your full attention, whether it's putting together an important presentation for work or taking out the trash. Pay attention to what is happening around you every second, but don't fight reality. If there is a long line at the post office or the DMV, accept it. After all, there's nothing you can do to speed things up. Instead, consider waiting in line a lesson in patience. Or use it as an opportunity to meditate or do a little people watching.

This is a lesson I wish I had learned earlier in life. Before my diagnosis, I was the master of multitasking. I had dozens of things on my plate at any one time as I managed two very demanding jobs, as well as family obligations. If you had asked me then, I would have proudly proclaimed that I accomplished this juggling act seamlessly. Little did I know that living in the moment is an even more effective way of managing work, not to mention life. I have discovered that by focusing on what I am doing in the moment, I not only gain more appreciation for the task at hand, I am also more productive and more present for those I am interacting with. We live in an age of distraction. Thousands of things beg for our attention every day. Living in the moment not only helps you live completely, it helps you to live with intention. You experience pleasures, both large and small, in ways you never have before.

There was a story I heard as a small boy about a man who was being chased toward the edge of a cliff by a tiger. At the bottom of the cliff was another tiger waiting for the man to jump. Surrounded by danger, the man leapt, grabbing a branch that was growing out of the rocky cliff wall. But the branch snapped under the man's weight, sending him hurtling toward certain death. Suddenly, he spied the most perfect strawberry he had ever seen. The man reached out and grabbed it. With mere seconds to live, he bit into the strawberry. As the juicy, flavorful berry burst in his mouth, he realized that it was the best strawberry he had ever eaten. In that moment, he was at peace. To me, this tale is the perfect example of living in the present.

In Japanese culture, the symbol of the cherry blossom is cherished because it is a metaphor for life. The bloom is intense, but fleeting. Savor your journey! What is the best way to start living in the moment? Try focusing on your breath. Become aware of what you are feeling right now. Just be.

Father and Sons

The hardest part of dealing with pancreatic cancer isn't the pain or the fact that I will, at some point, die. It is the sad certainty that I won't be able to watch my sons grow into the men I hope they will become.

I cried when I told James and Lane about the cancer. I cried because I knew that I would not be there for them. I cried—not because I fear death but because, as a father, I will be silenced. Telling my boys that I would not be around for them was the hardest thing I have ever done.

Amidst the tears, anger, and fear, my sons have had questions. I answer them as honestly and as completely as I can. My illness has made them grow up far too quickly, but I believe they will be stronger for it.

It's not all gloom and doom. It's important for all of us to build what good memories we can while I am still well enough to do so. And so we head to the stadium to cheer on the Washington Huskies every chance we get. Movies are also a family favorite. I've discovered that even the silliest comedy can offer opportunities to share a bit of wisdom with the kids. You can even find me in the kitchen with one or the other of the boys cooking up treats I am no longer allowed to eat. But it's the time spent together, not the cookies or cakes, that matters most.

The entire family is learning to seize the day—*carpe diem!* None of us know how many anniversaries Gwen and I will celebrate, or how many more of the boys' birthdays I will be able to share with them. It's not likely I'll be around for their college graduations and weddings. But we have today—and that's what counts.

The Three Ls

If you are living with cancer, it's easy to focus exclusively on your disease. But, it's important not to let cancer define you. I've found that concentrating on the following three things can help you cope, even on the bad days, and enhance your overall outlook.

LOVE. Surround yourself with the people and things you love. Follow your passions and spend time doing the things you love to do.

LIVE. Don't think of yourself as sick. Try to live as normal a life as you possibly can.

LAUGH. Have a happy life by concentrating on the positive. Smile!

CHAPTER FOUR

So Doc, What Are My Options?

It's not the load that breaks you down,
it's the way you carry it.
~ Lou Holtz

ECAUSE OF MY MEDICAL BACKGROUND, I knew I needed treatment, and fast. I wanted to know what my options were and how soon we could get started. While I was familiar with the major types of conventional cancer treatment, I didn't know which would be appropriate in my case. Dr. Saunders recommended that I meet with a surgeon and an oncologist as soon as possible. I asked him what type of treatment I could expect. He explained that, because my early-onset cancer is an aggressive disease, it often requires an aggressive approach. As I suspected, the protocols typically used to treat my cancer included chemotherapy, radiation, and surgery. Each has merit as well as drawbacks. It was just a matter of figuring out which treatments were right for me.

While I knew the basics of each type of treatment, Dr. Saunders gave me a quick review.

Chemotherapy

Chemotherapy is the use of specific drugs that are capable of killing cancer cells throughout the entire body. It can be a good option if cancer has metastasized.

More than 100 different chemo drugs exist and can be used in different combinations. The idea is that using several different drugs that have different actions can kill more cancer cells than using just one or two drugs. Combined therapy can also reduce the chance that the cancer may become resistant to any one chemo drug.

While combination chemo is used to treat a wide variety of cancers, the likely choice to treat ampulla or pancreatic cancer is gemcitabine HCl (trade name Gemzar). Gemcitabine is a single drug considered as a first-line treatment for patients with stage 2, 3, or 4 pancreatic cancer—and the one I assumed would be used in my case if my cancer was determined to be in the pancreas. It works by interfering with the process by which cells divide and repair themselves. This prevents the further growth of cancer cells and ultimately results in their death.

For some cancer patients, chemo may be the only treatment needed. More often, chemo is used along with surgery or radiation therapy (or both) to shrink a tumor. It can also kill any remaining cancer after surgery or radiation. When chemo is given after surgery, it is called adjuvant therapy. When it is used to shrink a tumor before surgery or radiation therapy, it is called neoadjuvant therapy.

The funny thing about chemo is that it essentially requires poisoning the body to save it. Healthy normal cells grow and divide in an orderly manner to replace old or damaged cells. Cancer cells have lost that capacity and they divide in an out-of-control manner. Chemotherapy drugs work by interfering with the ability of cancer cells to divide and reproduce themselves.

Each class of chemotherapy drugs damages cancer cells in different ways. Some prevent the cells from copying the key components they need to divide. Others either replace or eliminate essential enzymes or

---

Depending on the type of cancer and its stage, chemotherapy can be used to:

*   cure the cancer,
*   keep the cancer from spreading,
*   slow the cancer's growth,
*   kill cancer cells that may have spread to other parts of the body, and/or
*   relieve symptoms caused by cancer.

nutrients the cells need for their survival. Still others trigger cells to self-destruct in a process called apoptosis. The catch is that, if you overshoot the mark on the dosage of chemo drugs, the body might not be able to recover. When this happens, both the cancer cells and the healthy cells die. It's a delicate balancing act.

As you might expect, chemo comes with a host of side effects. When most people think of chemotherapy, they think of hair loss and nausea as the primary side effects. But depending on the strength and duration of your chemotherapy, the side effects of traditional treatment can also include anemia; constipation; diarrhea; fatigue; increased likelihood of bruising, bleeding, and infection; kidney and bladder irritation; muscle problems; nerve damage; reduced appetite and weight loss; sore mouth, gums, and throat; and sexual or fertility problems. Of course, not everyone experiences side effects. If they do, the severity can vary from person to person.

How often chemo is administered and how long treatment lasts depend on the kind of cancer, the goals of the treatment, the drugs being used, and how the body responds to them. Treatments may be given daily, weekly, or monthly, but they are usually given in on-and-off cycles. Taking a break from treatment periodically allows the body to build healthy new cells and regain its strength.

Radiation

Radiation therapy is a common way of treating solid tumors. About half of all people with pancreatic cancer receive radiation. Radiation can be administered by external beam therapy or internally using brachytherapy. Both methods break apart cancerous cells. Radiation also restores the cancer cell's innate ability to destroy itself.

There are different types of radiation and different ways to deliver it. For example, certain types of radiation can penetrate more deeply into the body than others. Some types of radiation can also be finely controlled to treat only a small area (an inch of tissue, for example) without damaging nearby tissues and organs. Other types of radiation are better suited for treating larger areas.

External beam radiation can be combined with surgery and/or chemotherapy to treat pancreatic cancer. It can also be used alone or with the chemotherapy drug gemcitabine for patients whose cancer is too

How Chemo Gets To Your Cancer Cells

Most chemo drugs are given intravenously through a tiny plastic tube called a catheter. The drugs can be given quickly through the catheter from a syringe over a few minutes. This is called an IV push. However, a typical IV infusion can last 30 minutes to a few hours. IVs aren't the only way chemotherapy drugs are given. Depending on the type of chemo drugs and where the cancer is located, your treatment may be administered in one of the following ways.

✳ **ORALLY.** You swallow the drug as a pill, capsule, or liquid just as you do other medicines. This is considerably more convenient because the drugs can be taken at home. If you take chemo drugs by mouth, it is important to take the exact dosage, at the right time, for as long as it has been prescribed for you.

✳ **INTRATHECAL.** The drug is put into the spinal canal and goes into the cerebrospinal fluid (the fluid that surrounds the brain and spinal cord). This is done either with a needle inserted directly into the spine, or with a long-term catheter and port surgically implanted under the scalp during surgery. This is called an Ommaya reservoir. The port is a small drum-like device that has a tiny tube attached to it. The tube goes in to the cerebrospinal fluid in the spinal canal. It stays in place under the skin until treatment is done.

✳ **INTRA-ARTERIAL.** The chemo drug is put directly into an artery. This can be used to treat a single area (such as an arm or leg), thus limiting the effect of the drug on other parts of the body.

✳ **INTRACAVITARY.** Chemo drugs may be given through a catheter into the abdominal cavity (the space around the bowels and other organs in the belly) or chest cavity (the space around the lungs and other organs in the chest).

✳ **INTRAMUSCULAR.** The drug is put into a muscle via injection (as a shot).

✳ **INTRALESIONAL.** A needle is used to put the drug directly into a tumor in the skin, under the skin, or in an internal organ.

✳ **TOPICAL.** The drug is put directly onto an area of cancer on the skin.

advanced to be removed surgically. When treating pancreatic cancer, the radiologist uses a high-energy X-ray machine called a linear accelerator to direct the radiation beams at the cancerous pancreatic tumor. It's a painless outpatient procedure that only lasts a few minutes and is typically given five days a week, over the course of six to eight weeks.

Some doctors prefer internal radiation for pancreatic cancer that has metastasized. In brachytherapy, the doctors place a source of radiation close to the tumor using hollow needles. This type of therapy may be used alone or in conjunction with external therapy. Unfortunately both types of radiation therapy damage neighboring cells, so side effects can occur. Many of these side effects—especially skin reactions—are directly related to the area being treated, but radiation can also cause fatigue and a loss of appetite. In some cases, it can lower white blood cell count, increasing susceptibility to infection.

Surgery

You might think that it makes sense to physically go in and remove the offending cancer and sometimes it does. Surgery for pancreatic cancer that hasn't spread can be very effective and can offer the best chance of extending survival. But this may not be the case if the cancer has metastasized to faraway sites in the body. If the tumor is too widespread to be completely removed, a surgeon may choose to do palliative surgery. Several studies show that simply removing part of the cancer without using any adjunct therapy like chemo or radiation does not help patients live longer. It can, however, relieve symptoms or prevent certain complications liked a blocked bile duct or intestinal tract. That said, GI surgery is no picnic. It is extremely invasive and complex, and recovery is very painful.

There are several types of surgery that can be used for patients with pancreatic cancer. The most common is the Whipple procedure, in which the head of the pancreas, part of the bile duct, the gallbladder, and the duodenum are typically removed. After these are removed, the remaining pancreas, bile duct, and intestine are sewn to the intestine so that gastrointestinal secretions flow back into the gut.

Other, less commonly used procedures include total pancreatectomy (in which the whole pancreas is removed, along with the gallbladder, part of the stomach, part of the small intestine, the bile duct, the spleen, and nearby lymph nodes) and distal pancreatectomy (in which the body and tail of the pancreas are removed). Both of these operations carry more risk and the outcome often isn't as successful as the Whipple procedure. That is one reason these surgeries aren't often used.

The Whipple Procedure

The Whipple operation was named after Dr. Allen Oldfather Whipple, the American surgeon who perfected the technique of resecting the pancreas, duodenum, and other organs in 1935. The Whipple performed today is very similar to the one performed back then—the biggest difference being safety. As recently as the 1960s and 1970s having a Whipple procedure carried a good deal of risk. In fact, up to 25 percent of patients died from the surgery. Fortunately, that has changed in recent years. A Whipple performed today by an experienced surgeon in a hospital in which large numbers of the procedure are performed carries less than 5 percent mortality risk.

The procedure's success depends on how far the cancer has spread. Overall, the 5-year survival rate after a Whipple operation is about 20 percent. If the cancer has not spread to the lymph nodes, the patient has a 40 percent chance of survival. Compare that to chemo alone at just 5 percent, and you can see how beneficial a Whipple operation can be for some people with pancreatic cancer.

The Whipple procedure can take four to six hours to complete. It is a very complex operation and complications can occur. These can include:

* **PANCREATIC FISTULA.** After the tumor is removed from the pancreas, the cut end of the pancreas is sewn to the intestine so pancreatic juices can travel back into the intestine. The pancreas is a very soft organ, and in some patients this suture line may not heal properly. If this happens, patients develop leakage of pancreatic juice. Usually the surgeon leaves behind a drainage catheter in the abdomen during the surgery. Any leakage of pancreatic juice after the surgery is usually removed from the body by this drainage catheter. In almost all patients who develop leakage of pancreatic juice after the surgery, the leakage heals on its own.

* **GASTROPARESIS (PARALYSIS OF THE STOMACH).** The first five to six days after the surgery, you will be provided with intravenous fluids until your

bowel function returns. After your bowel function has returned, your surgeon will begin you on a diet of clear liquids and your diet will progress to a regular diet as you tolerate it. However, some patients find that their stomach remains paralyzed after surgery. During this period you may not tolerate food very well. If you fall in this category, you will be provided with nutrition through a small feeding tube placed into the intestine at the time of surgery. In almost all patients, stomach function returns to normal within six weeks after surgery.

Surgery can also carry long-term consequences, including a diminished ability to absorb nutrients due to the reduced production of digestive enzymes. When this happens, patients can experience bulky, oily diarrhea. Long-term treatment with pancreatic enzyme supplements usually provides relief from this problem.

Smaller meals are also recommended after a Whipple to allow better absorption of food and to minimize feeling bloated or overly full. Because of this, it's not surprising for a patient to lose 5 to 10 percent of her body weight after surgery. This usually stabilizes after a few weeks, and most patients are able to maintain their weight and do well.

My Action Plan

Radiation was mentioned as a possible part of my therapy but soon discarded as an option since chemotherapy offered the best chance given the spread of my cancer. But first, I needed to have as much of the cancer removed as possible—and that meant a Whipple procedure to totally reconstruct my biliary tract, stomach, and small bowel. While I knew that the surgery wouldn't be a walk in the park, I also knew that,

---

You might need a Whipple if you have . . .

* Cancer of the head of the pancreas
* Cancer of the duodenum
* Cancer of the bottom end of the bile duct (cholangiocarcinoma)
* Cancer of the ampulla
* Benign tumors of the head of the pancreas
* Chronic pancreatitis (inflammation of the pancreas)

combined with the chemo, it was my best shot. After hearing my options, I decided on the surgery first while my body was strong enough to survive it. After the Whipple, I could rely on the chemotherapy to clean up any remaining cancer cells.

Picking the right surgeon to perform the procedure was critical. For a complex surgery like the Whipple procedure that had more connections and exits than the Santa Monica freeway, the skill of the surgeon would be paramount. Recent studies from Johns Hopkins and Memorial Sloan Kettering have shown that the outcome for a Whipple depends on the experience of the hospital and the surgeon performing the operation. In those hospitals that perform a large number of Whipples, the fatality rate is now less than 5 percent. But hospitals that don't perform many Whipples have a much higher rate of complications and death—often

---

の

A SPOUSE'S PERSPECTIVE: Waiting to Exhale

Mark's surgeon, Dr. Sinanan, entered the family waiting room to briefly describe the procedure and the estimated timeline. He also reassured us that he would take good care of Mark. He then left, only to return with an armload of blankets and pillows. This compassionate gesture could have been easily assigned to any staff member, but the doctor took this responsibility upon himself. He was caring for us as well as Mark, but it was a sure sign that we were in for a long night.

As midnight approached, Mark's mother Betty, my sister Fay, and I became the sole occupants of the hushed, dimly lit waiting room. Throughout the small hours of the morning, the three of us waited for the communal waiting room telephone to periodically ring. When we answered, a nurse's calm voice on the other end provided surgical updates on Mark's status and answered our questions.

We were exhausted but couldn't sleep. Our restless worries kept us on edge. This risky surgery that routinely takes six hours took much, much longer. At last, Dr. Sinanan appeared. I grabbed my pen and pad, ready to take notes. I knew Mark would want all the details.

The doctor told us that he had successfully removed and resected all the affected pieces and parts in Mark's digestive tract. Then he dropped the bombshell. It turned out that the ampulla cancer was far more widespread than they originally thought. It had

greater than 15 percent. So finding the right surgeon could very well be a matter of life or death.

Of course, anyone facing a critical surgery wants the very best. But finding the right surgeon can be easier said than done. Just asking your doctor won't necessarily yield the perfect referral. Most doctors avoid siding with one surgeon or specialist over another as a professional courtesy. Instead, I asked Dr. Saunders who he would go to if he had a family member who needed a Whipple. The answer was Mika Sinanan, MD, PhD, a Seattle-based surgeon who specializes in gastrointestinal surgery, particularly for patients with gastrointestinal cancers and pancreatic diseases. Luckily, Dr. Sinanan was able to fit me into his schedule. Two weeks later, I checked into the University of Washington Medical Center, ready to attack this evil thing inside of me.

---

spread into Mark's pancreas. As a result, 40 percent of the pancreas was very hard and had to be removed. "Like wood," explained the surgeon. He also had to remove the gall bladder and a one-foot section of Mark's colon. The rebuilding process involved restructuring the biliary tract and the stomach.

Fear gripped me as I looked down at my notes. Our family was all too familiar with pancreatic cancer—it was ruthless and deadly. We had watched the brutal suffering of loved ones who had courageously battled the disease. If you had to have cancer, this is the last type of cancer you would want.

My voice shook as I asked the surgeon, "What happens now?" Dr. Sinanan said that he thought he had removed 99 percent of the cancer. Chemotherapy would target the last one percent.

The next question was more difficult. "We have two sons. How do I tell them this is happening to their father? What words do I use?"

"I'm so sorry," he replied softly. It was the only answer Dr. Sinanan couldn't provide.

When he had left the room, three shattered women remained. Betty and Fay's shocked and frightened expressions mirrored my own. As we embraced, I thought of the heartbreaking task that lay ahead. I would need to give Mark and our sons the bad news.

— Gwen

Dr. Sinanan prefers to do his Whipple surgeries during the "grave-yard" shift. Here's why: Since a Whipple procedure can take at least six hours to complete, it can keep an operating room tied up for a good chunk of time. By scheduling my surgery in the wee hours, it wouldn't compete with other surgical needs. I just hoped this graveyard time frame wasn't a predictor of events to come.

Recovery Begins

I awoke to find myself in a hospital bed in the intensive care unit (ICU). Through my anesthesia-induced grogginess, I gradually became aware of the ventilator that was taped securely to my nose. It ran down my throat and into my stomach, making it impossible to speak. It occurred to me that the device, technically known as a nasogastric tube, must have made me look like some sort of distorted elephant. I certainly felt like one. There was an odd heaviness about me that I couldn't explain.

Gwen was stealing a few hours of sleep at home after what I would later learn was a grueling night in the waiting room, but I was not alone. My mother and sister Patti hovered near my bed. I motioned to them that I wanted to write a message. Somehow they understood and gave me a pen and paper. Dazed and shaky from the anesthesia, I tried to write a simple question: "How did the surgery go?" From their concerned faces, I could tell that the news wasn't good. But I wouldn't get the details until Gwen arrived a short time later.

Gwen looked tired when she walked into my room, even though she tried not to show it. Instead, she smiled broadly and asked me how I felt. She slipped her hand underneath my palm, being careful not to dislodge the IV taped to the back of my hand. But the sad, gentle look in her eyes confirmed my suspicions that things had not gone well. She slowly explained that the cancer had spread through much of my pancreas, as well as my colon, chest, and neck. I immediately thought of Uncle Nobi, who had passed away from unrelenting pancreatic cancer just months earlier. I was sure that my wife, mother, and sister were afraid that I was heading down the same path. I was afraid, too.

I had to get well. I simply had to. I had too many responsibilities, too many things left to do. I wasn't about to let cancer cut short my time on this earth. I knew that I needed to heal from my surgery as soon as possible so I could begin chemotherapy. While a typical Whipple recovery can drag on for months, I didn't think that I had the luxury of time. If I could get on top of this cancer before it began to flourish again, I might have a fighting chance. Fortunately—although I didn't know it at the time—the stars aligned to help speed things along.

No Pain, No Gain?

The pain from my six-inch incision began to make itself known the next day. I was given a pain pump that would dispense morphine at the press of a button, and I was told to use the maximum amount to provide comfort. But I had a better idea. Because I was so determined to have a quick recovery, I intentionally refrained from using my pain pump unless absolutely necessary, essentially cutting the dose to about a quarter of what I needed. There was a method to my madness. My pharmacy background told me that narcotics like morphine can slow down gastrointestinal (GI) function. Since this would delay my recovery, I figured that I would put up with a little pain in exchange for a functioning GI tract. It sounded great in theory, but it certainly wasn't very effective in practice.

It turns out that the Whipple procedure is notorious for causing gastroparesis. I found myself in pain and with a stomach that was paralyzed. I couldn't eat and nothing I did would change things. It would be six long weeks before my food would come from something other than an IV tube.

Between the pain and the fact that I had just had my entire insides rearranged, I had hoped that the nurses would cut me some slack and let me rest for a day or two. No dice. Every hospital and every doctor does things a little differently after a Whipple, but one thing is the same: You walk, and the sooner the better. Walking helps with all aspects of recovery. It also helps prevent blood clots.

The day after surgery, I found myself bent over with pain as I shuffled down the hallway, my IV poles and multiple drain bags trailing behind me. One of the nurses offered encouraging words as she accompanied me every short, painful step of the way. I didn't get far during that first trip—to the nurses' station and back. Yet that was just the first of five daily walks I was required to take. Over the next few days, I began to look forward to my hallway strolls, especially the 2 a.m. jaunts. The hallways were relatively quiet then, and I could open my throttle up all the way. Before long, I was circling the nurses' station at a brisk clip of 100 feet per hour.

I soon discovered that nothing is quite as uncomfortable as a hospital bed, and walking gave me a chance to work the kinks out of my back. I also realized that ICUs are not set up to ensure a good night's sleep. If you are lucky, you are able to doze briefly between the seemingly continuous visits from lab techs, respiratory therapists, and nurses. But I was making progress. My recovery was on track, largely due to the efforts of remarkable staff of doctors, residents, and nurses. Dr. Sinanan was the

---

A SPOUSE'S PERSPECTIVE: The Pep Talk

For months, Mark's days had been filled with pain, infections, restrictive diets, sleepless nights, doctor appointments, blood tests, CT scans, MRIs, surgical procedures, and an unimaginable recovery process. It seemed like every time he made a little bit of progress, something would send him reeling backward. And while he did his best to keep his "game face" on, there were days when he wavered. It was understandable. I don't know if I could have faced what Mark did with the incredible amount courage he had.

I thought Mark would be in good spirits during his last day in the ICU. But, as I packed up Mark's things in anticipation of a move to the surgical recovery floor, I noticed that he seemed quiet and more than a little exhausted. Fortunately, someone "up there" was getting ready to throw Mark a much-needed bone.

Once Mark was ready for the move, I slipped out to use the restroom. As I headed down the ICU hallway, I thought about the emotional roller coaster we found ourselves on and prayed for the strength to deal with whatever lay ahead. As I approached the bathroom, I passed a familiar face. The man was pacing the hallway as he looked up at me and smiled. Who was this mystery man? I could swear I knew him. And then it hit me: He was the former coach of Mark's favorite football team, the University of Washington Huskies.

"Aren't you Jim Lambright?" I asked without hesitation. "Yes, I am," he replied, seemingly surprised that anyone recognized him in this setting. He had been patiently waiting for a group of very chatty doctors, residents, and nurses to vacate his wife's ICU room. It didn't seem like that would happen anytime soon, so I took the opportunity to strike up a conversation.

most amazing of all. Despite an incredibly full schedule, he managed to visit me every day to follow my post-op progress. Some days, he wouldn't make it until late in the day; there would be a knock on the door after 9:00 p.m., and he would poke his head into my room to check on me.

The care a surgeon gives goes well beyond the operating room—or at least it should. Dr. Sinanan made me feel like he was just as committed to my recovery as I was. One day shortly after my surgery, I was scheduled

---

꩜

"We are huge fans of yours and the Husky football team," I said. Then, summoning up my courage, I steamrolled ahead. "I don't mean to intrude, but if you have a few minutes, can you meet my husband?" I quickly brought the coach up to speed on Mark's condition. With nothing but a heart of gold, and time on his hands, Coach smiled and said, "Sure. What's his name?"

We found Mark sitting in the shadows, staring into space. The only light came from the TV. I pulled back the curtain and said, "Mark, there's a friend here who wants to see you."

"Hi Mark! How are you doing?"

It took Mark a few seconds to realize who was standing in front of him. This was the last person he expected to see in the ICU. His surprise quickly turned to delight.

"Hi Coach," he stammered. "Um, I've been sidelined."

The coach sat on the edge of Mark's bed and eyed one of the bile drainage bags that dangled from his chair. "That's a nice green color you've got there," he joked. Then he explained that he had once had one of those bags, too. "My wife and I are both kidney cancer survivors. When my doctors first gave me the news, I told them that I was too busy to have cancer. I had too many things that I still needed to do."

The coach leaned a little closer and told Mark, "I also told them that I don't lose, damn it! You need to tell your doctors the same thing!" Then Coach Lambright lightly tapped Mark's left knee with his fist to emphasize his point. Mark beamed.

While it may have been a small act on the coach's part, it was just the pep talk Mark needed. It was a simple gesture to emphasize the simple fact that you can't win if you don't fight. We will forever be grateful.

— Gwen

to have an abdominal CT scan to check my progress. I was sitting on the edge of my hospital bed waiting for a nurse to wheel me down to radiology. The next thing I knew, Dr. Sinanan was pushing a wheelchair through the door to personally escort me to my scan. This was truly above and beyond the call of duty! His unfailing attention helped keep me focused on getting better, even on the days when I was sick of the pain, sick of not sleeping, sick of being poked and prodded, and sick of being sick.

The Importance of Attitude

All the brilliant surgeons and cutting-edge medicine in the world can only do so much if the patient isn't motivated to get well. I was highly motivated, but I also had a lot of help. During the three weeks I was in the hospital, family members were my constant companions. My mother became a permanent fixture during the nightshift, sleeping in a lounge chair next to my bed and attending to my every need. I told her that she didn't need to do this, but it's a mother's right to hold a vigil for her child. To be fair, if James or Lane were in my situation, I would exercise my parental nightshift rights, too.

The dayshift was handled by Gwen and her incredibly supportive sister Fay. When Gwen and Fay needed a break, our friend Klari and my cousin Ed would take turns keeping watch over me.

My sister Patti was also a frequent visitor. A courageous breast cancer survivor, she provided me with untold inspiration. My other sister Terri, although out of town, sent countless card and letters, all with uplifting and encouraging messages.

Phone calls and visitors were restricted so that I could conserve my strength. We relied on my work colleague, Philip Olufson—considered "a brother from another mother"—to manage communications. But, even though contact was limited, I was bolstered by the avalanche of cards I received from family, friends, and coworkers. At one point, I looked at Gwen and said, "How can I not get better with all of these people praying for me?"

All of these prayers and well-wishes simply reinforced my determination to make a strong and quick recovery. If there was anything in my power I could do to hasten my recuperation and start chemotherapy, I was willing to give it a try. I was in a race for my life to find the right chemotherapy regimen. It was a race I simply couldn't lose.

CHAPTER FIVE

A Different Point of View

*The key to success is to risk thinking unconventional
thoughts. Convention is the enemy of progress.
If you go down just one corridor of thought you
never get to see what's in the rooms leading off it.*
~ *Trevor Baylis*

THE GOOD NEWS WAS THAT Dr. Sinanan thought he had gotten almost all the cancer during the Whipple procedure. He had hopes that chemotherapy would target any remaining cancer cells. The bad news was that the cancer had spread farther than anyone had originally thought. It was a killer diagnosis—stage 4 pancreatic cancer. Very few people get well from a diagnosis like this.

Still, I was determined to fight this devastating disease. My wife, my mom, and my sisters had stuck by me throughout the tests, the surgery, and the days when I could barely function. I wasn't going to bail on them now.

As my body recuperated from the Whipple operation, Gwen and I wondered if my body could survive the trials of chemotherapy. A month earlier, we had handpicked my oncologist from the many talented doctors in the Seattle area. Seattle is a cancer center of excellence with many fine oncologists to choose from. But I knew this was a critical choice since chemotherapy would be a key part of my post-surgery treatment. I would probably be spending a lot of time with my oncologist, so it was essential that he or she and I "clicked."

I had assumed that I would be seeing a conventional oncologist and that I would be given gemcitabine—a conventional chemo drug often used in cases of pancreatic cancer. Study after study has found that gemcitabine, used either by itself or combined with one or two other chemo drugs, offered the best chance of survival—at least for vast majority of pancreatic cancer patients whose bodies are receptive to the drug. A small number of people have a glitch in their genes that makes them resistant to gemcitabine. I hoped I wasn't one of them.

To complicate chemotherapy treatment options, there was a possibility that the cancer hadn't originated in my pancreas. According to the operative biopsy report, the cancer may have actually started in the small bowel. My dire prognosis remained dim no matter the area of origin of the cancer because of its widespread presence in my pancreas, ampulla, billiary tract, small bowel, colon, and distant lymph nodes. What did matter was how the cancer would be approached. Traditionally, gemcitabine would be the primary chemotherapy agent for treating pancreatic cancer. However, it might not be the best option if the origin was the small bowel. But which chemotherapy drugs would best target both types of cancer? All of those decisions and the ultimate direction my therapy would take would depend largely on the oncologist I ended up choosing to help me attack the beast within me.

Finding the right oncologist can be an intense process. It requires a lot of research. Typically, people start by asking their doctor for referrals to oncologists who specialize in the type of cancer they have. It's important to find oncologists who are covered by your insurance plan, too. The Internet has also become a useful tool when looking for a doctor. Web sites like UCompare HealthCare (www.ucompare-healthcare.com) and HealthGrades (www.healthgrades.com) offer information on the qualifications of specific doctors, as well as patient reviews. But perhaps the best way to find the right doctor for you is through referrals from family and friends. This is ultimately how I found Ben Chue, MD.

A Twist of Fate

Gwen dashed into the house one morning with the newspaper in her hand. "Look, Mark!" she said as she excitedly pointed to the front page. "Isn't this the doctor who treated Mindy's mom?" I looked at the caption underneath the photo of a man about my age. *Dr. Ben Chue.* Yes, the name did sound familiar. And then I remembered.

Several months earlier, I had flown into Southern California's John Wayne Orange County airport for a pharmaceutical conference. One of the perks my job provided was the opportunity to periodically escape the wet and dreary Washington weather and travel to warmer, drier climates. This was one such trip. I was anxious to get out of the airport and soak up some warm California sunshine. As I impatiently waited for my luggage to appear in baggage claim, my cell phone rang. It was one of my very best friends, Sandy Salzberg. After a few pleasantries, I asked him how his wife, Mindy, and her mother were doing. Mindy's mom had been diagnosed with an especially aggressive cancer.

Sandy mentioned that Mindy had found a wonderful oncologist named Dr. Ben Chue. He also said that Dr. Chue was a bit of a maverick. Apparently, he used unconventional chemotherapy combinations and worked with an acupuncturist, as well as a naturopath who specialized in oncology. But what really got my attention was when Sandy told me that Dr. Chue was actively looking for terminally ill patients with stage 4 pancreatic cancer. *Wow,* I remember thinking, *this guy sure sounds confident. Maybe a little too confident.*

As I pulled my mind back to the present, I looked at the article in front of me. It told the story of a 35-year-old pancreatic cancer patient named Aaron who had run out of conventional treatment options. Because he had been young and strong, Aaron's body had been blasted with the highest dose of chemo possible—two weeks on and two weeks off. But it hadn't worked. Instead, his feet became so swollen they looked like footballs, his thinking became cloudy, and he suffered from internal bleeding. After a stint in the intensive care unit because of a bad reaction from a blood transfusion, Aaron was out of options, according to his doctors.

With nothing left to lose, he turned to Dr. Chue. This young man was literally on death's doorstep as he was wheeled into Seattle Cancer Treatment and Wellness Center—but he wasn't there to die. He fully intended to live. Fortunately, Dr. Chue was up for the challenge.

The new treatment was based on standard chemotherapy agents, but in unique combinations. It also used lower doses and was given more frequently. The theory behind this approach is that it provides more chemotherapy over time, which increases its effectiveness. And, because the doses are lower, it potentially reduces unpleasant side effects like nausea and vomiting.

The article went on to say that this type of chemotherapy, also called dose-density or metronomic treatment, had shown some success in trials with lung and breast cancer patients. At the time, there were no studies on this novel approach for pancreatic cancer, especially such advanced cancer. This would be a first. But along with the unconventional chemo treatment, Aaron would also receive the controversial addition of a customized diet, targeted supplements, and lifestyle care from an oncology naturopath.

It worked. Two and a half years after meeting Dr. Chue, Aaron was virtually cancer-free. An avid biker, he was well enough to ride again and, at the time of the article, was training to compete in the Seattle-to-Portland Bicycle Classic.

Hmmm, I thought. *Maybe this Dr. Chue is on to something.* Turning back to the article, I noticed that Dr. Chue was recruiting for a phase-two clinical trial. Could he help me, too?

Thanks to my medical background, I knew what traditional chemotherapy could and could not do. If I opted for conventional therapy, the prognosis might just buy me a few more weeks or months. Dr. Chue's chemo protocol, on the other hand, could help me live much longer, if it worked—or shorten it, if it didn't.

If I had been talking to someone with my prognosis, I would have told them to go the conventional route. After all, it's proven and considered the "gold standard" for cancer. And yet, I couldn't get the idea of this new type of therapy out of my head. Apparently, I wasn't the only one. My cousin Eric had also seen the article and had passed it on to me via e-mail with a note urging me to check it out.

Throughout my life, I've found that when opportunity keeps knocking at your door, it's wise to at least open the door and see what is on the other side. In this case, it was Dr. Chue's unorthodox cancer treatment. It was outside of my evidence-based medical training, but it intrigued me—even though it didn't have volumes of research backing it up. I decided to take a chance.

While Gwen was on board with my decision, it shocked many of my friends and colleagues. I've always been very adverse to risk, so they assumed I would opt for standard treatment. The desire for more time with my family, more time to live, swayed me in a direction that surprised even me. I chose Dr. Chue and his unconventional chemotherapy treatment. It has been one of the best decisions I have ever made.

A Different Path

Once I had decided to take this leap of faith, I called to make an appointment with Dr. Chue. Even if I wasn't totally sold, what did I have to lose? If this nonconformist approach worked, I might buy myself years instead of months. But getting in to see the doctor proved more difficult than I had imagined. Thanks to his recent celebrity, Dr. Chue was booked solid. Patients from all over the country flocked to see him. His office said that we might be able to meet with one of his associates sometime in the future, but Gwen was insistent. After explaining my situation, Gwen managed to secure what would prove to be a life-changing appointment with Dr. Chue himself.

That first appointment really opened my eyes to how different Dr. Chue's treatment would be. His honesty was refreshing, even though he stressed that, since the cancer had spread to my neck, chest, and abdomen, he couldn't promise miracles. He was also the one doctor who noted that, while pancreatic cancer was the treatment focus, there was a chance I had cancer of the small bowel based on the operative biopsy of my ampulla. As I already mentioned, this could—and ultimately did—affect the treatment plan, which resulted in a course of action that targeted both the pancreas and the small bowel.

Dr. Chue spent the next two and a half hours answering our many questions. I asked about his philosophy and about the benefits I could expect from the combination of integrative oncology, naturopathy, and acupuncture. I also wanted to see the evidence, especially when it came to metronomic dosing. His answers astounded me. Unlike conventional chemotherapy, Dr. Chue's approach didn't have volumes of peer-reviewed evidence to back it up and yet it made complete sense. And, unlike traditional treatment, it appeared to trigger far fewer side effects.

I was in. I asked the only question that hadn't been asked—"How soon can we get started?"

Choices in Chemo

Chemotherapy is like a buffet dinner: There are lots of choices that can be combined in any number of ways. In traditional chemotherapy there are set protocols, which means certain drugs are typically used in certain combinations. It's predictable, like a traditional dinner—you start with your salad, followed by the entrée, and finish with dessert. For pancreatic cancer, you would start with gemcitabine and add on certain chemo drugs in a precise order as you move through the line. Cancer of the small bowel requires different chemotherapy drugs, but these drugs are also used according to a set protocol.

Dr. Chue doesn't limit himself to these predetermined protocols or established doses. Instead, he is willing to strategically sequence and customize chemo drugs depending on the patient's individual needs. If chemo was a buffet, Dr. Chue might start you with dessert. You might also find that the combinations on your plate don't conform to tradition either.

In both standard and metronomic chemotherapy, the drugs used work by damaging the DNA in cancer cells and disrupting their ability to replicate. Traditionally this is done by using specific combinations of these drugs at the highest possible dose to kill the most cancer cells without killing the patient. This is known as the "maximum tolerated dose," or MTD. A standard chemotherapy regimen could be just one or up to three weeks of treatment with three weeks of rest to allow the body to recover. While this approach can work, nearly half of all cancer patients eventually become resistant to the chemo drugs and succumb to their disease.

If chemotherapy doesn't kill you, the side effects can be considerable during your treatment—whether you opt for conventional chemo or go for a less traditional approach. It all depends on how your body handles the drugs. If your body has been weakened by the disease, you may be more vulnerable.

Side effects can have a significant impact on whether or not you will be able to tolerate and complete the therapy. In my experience, the aggressive treatment regimen that I was given resulted in many side effects, but the intensity was muted by the metronomic dosing patterns. Although the body blows associated with chemotherapy can vary depending on the drugs and doses used, here are the most common:

✻ **ANEMIA.** Chemotherapy doesn't just attack cancer cells. It can also attack healthy red blood cells and negatively impact the body's ability to produce more of them. A lack of red blood cells can cause anemia. Anemia is one of the most common and most lasting side effects of chemotherapy. In fact, seven out of 10 cancer patients experience anemia during chemo. I was one of them. My chemo-related anemia contributed to a feeling of fatigue when I over-exerted myself. Fortunately, I was able to muster up enough stamina to continue working during my chemotherapy.

While anemia places extra demands on the body and can cause excessive fatigue that can interfere with everyday activities, it can also cause dizziness, headaches, diminished sex drive, and a rapid heartbeat. Some people may also experience an inability to concentrate, paleness, and shortness of breath.

* **"CHEMO BRAIN."** This phrase is often used by cancer patients to describe changes in their memory, attention span, ability to concentrate, and ability to perform various mental tasks after they begin receiving chemotherapy treatments. High-dose chemotherapy appears to put patients at more risk of short-term memory loss and difficulty concentrating than metronomic dosing. In some cancer survivors, cognitive function can be impaired for years after chemo has ended.

As I headed into chemotherapy, this was of great concern for me. My brain is on overload as a standard of practice and I couldn't afford to diminish its function. Although I did experience some concentration challenges, I managed to push through the mental fog.

* **EDEMA.** Some chemotherapy drugs can cause fluid retention in the body. This form of swelling is most noticeable in the feet, ankles, hands, and face. Ascites is a related problem in which abnormal amounts of fluid collect in the stomach or abdomen. Symptoms of ascites include swelling or puffiness of the abdomen or stomach, tight or shiny skin over the stomach, feeling full sooner than normal during meals, and being able to see the veins on the skin of the abdomen. Fortunately, edema usually subsides once chemotherapy drugs are stopped.

* **HAIR LOSS.** By the fourth week of chemotherapy, my hair loss was significant. I began shedding like a dog and I was bald by week six. Hair loss occurs because chemotherapy affects all the cells in the body. The lining of the mouth and stomach, as well as hair follicles, are especially sensitive because those cells multiply rapidly just like the cancer cells. The difference is that the normal cells will repair themselves, making these side effects temporary. While hair loss can be one of the most emotionally distressing side effects, the good news is that hair loss does not occur with all types of chemotherapy. Whether or not your hair remains as it is, thins, or falls out depends on the drugs and dosages used.

* **IMMUNOSUPPRESSION.** This was one of the most challenging side effects of my chemotherapy. As chemotherapy kills cancer cells, it also negatively affects white blood cells that are responsible for fighting off infection. If white blood cell counts drop to perilously low levels, a serious, life-threatening infection can result. The hit to my immune system was severe enough to require white blood cell booster shots to my stomach, which Gwen bravely administered. A nutrient-dense diet and immune-boosting supplements can also help prevent infection and illness during chemotherapy.

* **NAUSEA, DIARRHEA, AND VOMITING.** These gastrointestinal symptoms can be among the most debilitating side effects of chemotherapy. They not only affect a patient's desire to continue treatment, they can interfere with the ability to consume a nutritious diet. This can lead to weight loss and malnutrition. Certain chemotherapy drugs are more likely than are others to cause nausea and vomiting. Whether a drug will cause nausea and vomiting also depends on the dosage. Some drugs may be less likely to cause side effects at lower dosages. I believe this is where the metronomic dosing shines. While I did experience nausea, it was never so severe that I vomited.

Other factors can also determine risk. Women, people under the age of 50, teetotalers, and people with a high level of anxiety are more likely to suffer gastrointestinal issues. In addition, the expectation that treatment will cause nausea and vomiting increases the chances that it will. Some patients even experience anticipatory nausea and vomiting triggered by certain sights and smells associated with chemotherapy. Driving by their chemotherapy center or seeing their oncologist can trigger waves of nausea or worse. One story recounted for me involved a patient who, by chance, ran into her oncologist at the supermarket. Upon seeing him, the patient began to vomit uncontrollably. This just reinforces the impact the mind can have on the body.

* **PERIPHERAL NEUROPATHY.** Certain chemotherapy drugs can damage nerve endings, resulting in numbness, burning, and severe pain in the extremities—especially hands and feet. This can make it extremely difficult, or even impossible, to perform normal activities like walking, driving, typing, picking up objects, and even eating. The severity and duration of the neuropathy can vary, but because the nerve endings are damaged, it can become a chronic condition that persists long after the chemotherapy has ended.

The chemotherapy regimen that I was on produced significant neuropathy. It became so severe that walking was difficult and driving, impossible. Fortunately, thanks to time, supplements, and medication, I am now back in the driver's seat and walk regularly on a treadmill. What's more, I can again button my dress shirts and tie my necktie—even though Gwen still has to make sure they coordinate.

* **THROMBOCYTOPENIA.** Many chemotherapy drugs temporarily stop cells from dividing—especially the cells that divide quickly like red and white blood cells and platelets, which are made by bone marrow. This can not only lower blood and platelet counts, it can affect the ability of the blood to clot normally, which puts the patient at risk of excessive bleeding.

A low platelet count typically occurs six to 10 days after the administration of chemotherapy and continues for several days. Infrequently, cancer patients may also experience thrombocytopenia from other medications or as a consequence of their underlying cancer.

If your platelet count is low, you should try to avoid situations that may cause injury, bruising, or bleeding. Do only low-impact activity for exercise, such as walking or swimming. Shave with an electric razor instead of a blade, and use a soft-bristle toothbrush.

Thrombocytopenia is a perfect example of the power of naturopathic oncology. Conventional medicine isn't able to provide medication that will boost platelet counts. However, under the guidance of my naturopathic oncologist, I took a daily dose of unrefined cold-pressed—not processed or toasted—sesame oil. While this approach does not work for everyone, I was lucky to be a responder. This resulted in a return to normal platelet counts. This miraculous rise in platelets meant that I was able to continue with uninterrupted chemotherapy doses.

While some of these side effects can be treated with conventional medications, they can be a real problem for anyone undergoing maximum dose chemotherapy. Fortunately, personalized chemotherapy combinations paired with low dosing can minimize uncomfortable and potentially life-threatening side effects. I know they have worked extremely well for me.

Less Is More

What I found even more fascinating than Dr. Chue's personalized chemo combinations was the way he approached dosing. Most oncologists believe that stronger doses, using the MTD, are the most effective way to battle cancer cells. But chemotherapy pioneers like Dr. Chue are finding success with the continuous use of low doses of chemotherapy drugs. This novel approach is proving so effective that some researchers think it may be the key to making cancer a chronic, manageable disease instead of a potential killer. It also offers hope to those who have run out of conventional options.

Mainstream chemo targets cancer cells with massive doses of highly toxic drugs that are given for a limited period of time—typically one to three weeks—followed by a rest period to allow normal tissue to recover. The problem is that this "timeout" allows tumor cells to mutate and become drug-resistant. The tiny blood vessels that nourish the cancer cells also flourish during these rest periods. Tumor growth depends on this blood supply, which is one reason that simply targeting tumors often fails. When the patient becomes resistant to the chemotherapy agents being used, the tumor thrives thanks to a healthy network of blood vessels.

Low-dose or metronomic dosing relies on the continuous use of chemo drugs, but at doses far below what is normally used—sometimes as low as one-tenth the conventional dose. By eliminating the rest periods, metronomic dosing not only kills some cancer cells directly, but also prevents the formation of new blood vessels that feed any remaining tumor cells.

This isn't a new concept. For years, pediatric oncologists have successfully used constant low-dose chemotherapy in kids with leukemia. And studies conducted at Memorial Sloan-Kettering Cancer Center show that low-dose chemotherapy has shrunk or stabilized tumors in up to three-quarters of women with breast cancer, 60 percent of patients with lung cancer, 50 percent of children with brain cancer, and 30 percent of women with ovarian cancer.

Encouraged by these findings, Dr. Chue reasoned that the low-dose approach would also be effective for people with pancreatic cancer who had developed a resistance to conventional chemotherapy. By the time I saw him, Dr. Chue had successfully treated seven late-stage pancreatic cancer patients who had been given up for dead by their conventional oncologists. Even though I was a chemotherapy novice, Dr. Chue's approach made sense from the outset.

Perhaps the biggest advantage to metronomic dosing from a patient's perspective is that side effects are more tolerable. Because the body isn't being blasted by large amounts of poison, there is reduced toxicity to white blood cells—which means less chance of infection. Patients also experience less nausea and vomiting.

Of course, metronomic dosing and unconventional chemo drug combinations are no guarantee that patients will avoid all side effects. To help manage these ill effects, Dr. Chue turns to naturopathy, Chinese herbal medicine, and acupuncture. While not utilized by most oncologists, these alternative healing methods are very familiar to Dr. Chue, who grew up in San Francisco's Chinatown, where herbal tonics based on Traditional Chinese Medicine (TCM) were widely used for colds, flu, and pain relief. He never forgot these traditional medicines, even as he studied at some of the country's most prestigious medical schools, including Yale and the University of California, San Francisco Medical School. Dr. Chue believes that this upbringing helped keep his mind open to other types of healing.

Combining this novel form of chemotherapy with herbal remedies, acupuncture, nutrition, stress relief, and other lifestyle changes is proving incredibly effective. While there aren't any studies that compare the survival statistics of Dr. Chue's patients to patients undergoing conventional treatment, it's clear that, even if this treatment doesn't extend life, it certainly enhances the quality of life. But, for me—I've found both quantity and quality because of my decision to try a new type of medicine.

Preparing for Battle

Getting one's body ready for chemotherapy is critical; it can help prevent debilitating side effects and can speed up recovery. I was told not to overdo it or wear myself out before I started treatment. It seems that many people facing chemo rush around trying to get everything in order before treatment begins. They assume that they will be too sick to do anything during and after treatment, so they exhaust themselves in the days and weeks before their treatment.

Fortunately, Gwen—with the help of our extended family—picked up the slack. She kept track of the house, the boys' schedules, and my never-ending medical appointments while making sure I followed doctor's orders. She also created "Team Mark" to keep family, friends, and coworkers apprised of my progress via e-mail. This allowed me to focus on getting ready for my upcoming chemotherapy.

Strengthening my body was critical. Along with getting plenty of sleep, I needed to change the way I was eating. Good nutrition is critical if you are undergoing chemotherapy. It's estimated that up to 80 percent of cancer patients are malnourished. But, it turns out that people who eat well before and during chemotherapy tend to have fewer side effects. They also are more likely to complete the full course of therapy than those who are poorly nourished.

I wanted to do everything I could to be able to finish my therapy, so I traded in my burgers and pizza for fresh fruits and vegetables, whole grains, and lots of low-fat protein. Large amounts of high-quality protein

METRONOMIC VS. CONVENTIONAL THERAPY		
TREATMENT WEEK	**CONVENTIONAL DOSING**	**METRONOMIC DOSING**
1	10	5
2		5
3		5
4	10	5
5		5
6		5
7	10	5
8		5
9		5
10	10	5
11		5
12		5
Total Dose Weeks 1 to 12	**40**	**60**

are particularly important for people undergoing chemotherapy because protein is essential for repairing the tissue damage that occurs during the treatments. In fact, people undergoing chemo should aim to consume about 80 grams of protein daily—nearly twice the amount that healthy adults need. Cancer patients who increase their protein about a week before chemotherapy and continue to consume extra protein afterward recover more quickly. They also have more energy and less fatigue. Along with fish, skinless poultry, beans, and nuts, an easy way to add protein is to drink smoothies made with fresh or frozen fruit like blueberries and strawberries, a scoop of whey protein powder that provides 15 to 22 gm of protein per serving, and a tablespoon of flax seed meal. Not only will this pump up protein intake, it is a good source of fiber and fruit-derived bioflavonoids.

Chemo-Time

Chemotherapy—especially the way it would be administered by Dr. Chue—made sense to me. I knew it was my best shot. But I was also

---

Pass the Mustard

Have you ever wondered how chemotherapy came into being? Oddly enough, it didn't start out as a way to kill cancer. Instead, it was a biological agent of war designed to kill soldiers.

During World War I, mustard gas was a key chemical weapon. After an accidental exposure of a group of soldiers during World War II, researchers discovered that the men who were exposed to mustard gas had low white blood cell counts. They reasoned that an agent with such an effect on rapidly dividing white blood cells might also have the same effect on cancer cells. Autopsies showed that people exposed to mustard gas had also experienced the suppression of two types of white blood cells: lymphoids and myeloids. Based on these discoveries, a form of intravenous mustard gas was given to individuals with late-stage lymphomas. The results were dramatic: Their improvement, although temporary, was remarkable.

Through the years, other research has helped to discover many more chemotherapeutic agents to treat cancer. Today, treatment is far more focused and effective than in those early days, but the basic principles and limitations of the therapy still remain.

a bit nervous as I approached this new experience. The word "chemo-therapy" carries such an ominous aura, thanks largely to books, movies, and TV shows portraying the therapy as a fate worse than death. It's no wonder cancer patients are fearful of the treatments.

As I walked into Dr. Chue's office at the Seattle Cancer Treatment and Wellness Center on that first day of my weekly chemo treatments, I felt like I was as prepared as I could be. I had done everything asked of me in anticipation of my upcoming chemo.

I also knew exactly what I was getting myself into. I had given Dr. Chue the third degree and he had graciously answered all of my

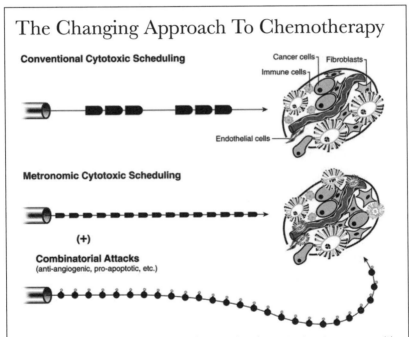

The Changing Approach To Chemotherapy

Conventional Cytotoxic Scheduling

Cancer cells
Fibroblasts
Immune cells
Endothelial cells

Metronomic Cytotoxic Scheduling

(+)

Combinatorial Attacks
(anti-angiogenic, pro-apoptotic, etc.)

The conventional logic of chemotherapy has been to treat cancers with closely spaced infusions of drugs at or near the maximum tolerable dose, followed by substantial rest periods. The typical results were temporary improvements in tumor growth and the extension of life-span. But it was also accompanied by disturbing side effects and eventual relapse. Metronomic chemotherapy involves constant dosing without rest periods using lower doses to minimize toxic side effects. Metronomic dosing and the use of targeted drug combinations can kill tumor cells as well as the endothelial cells in blood vessels. The bullets refer to doses of chemo-therapy, which can be large and episodic (upper picture) or smaller and metronomic (lower picture). The bombs in the bottom picture indicate other anticancer agents providing additive or synergistic benefits.

SOURCE: THE JOURNAL OF CLINICAL INVESTIGATION

questions. Being a pharmacist, I wanted to know all of the details—drugs, doses, expected outcomes, typical side effects. I was surprised when he told me that gemcitabine was not on the menu. Gemcitabine is used specifically to treat pancreatic cancer. But since there was a possibility that I might have small bowel cancer, Dr. Chue opted for a chemo cocktail of oxaliplatin, paclitaxel, leucovorin, and 5-fluorouracil that could target both types of cancer.

Like other platinum derivatives, oxaliplatin is classified as an alkylating agent and is commonly used to treat colon and rectal cancers that have metastasized. At typical doses used in conventional chemotherapy, oxaliplatin can trigger a laundry list of side effects including gastrointestinal problems, low blood counts, and especially peripheral neuropathy.

Paclitaxel is best known for its effect on breast cancer. It targets cancer cells and works by interfering with cell division. But this cancer-fighting action often comes at the cost of hair. And like oxaliplatin, it can trigger GI problems and peripheral neuropathy. Leucovorin, which is actually a reduced form of the B vitamin folic acid, is used to treat many types of gastrointestinal cancer. While not technically a chemotherapy drug, leucovorin helps to bind another anticancer drug 5-fluorouracil—to an enzyme inside of the cancer cells. As a bonus, it also helps reduce chemotherapy's side effects.

The final drug in my chemo combination was 5-fluorouracil, another chemo drug that hampers cell division. It can also negatively affect the GI tract, cause mouth sores, and send platelets and blood cell count south. 5-fluorouracil can also cause hand-foot syndrome (Palmar-Plantar Erythrodysesthesia), an eczema-like condition that triggers a rash, swelling, redness, pain, and/or peeling of the skin on the palms of hands and soles of feet.

While I knew the typical side effects people often experienced when taking these chemotherapy drugs at full dose, what I couldn't anticipate was how my own body would react to having these poisons injected into it, even at a lower dose. Before I would have a chance to find out, however, a lab technician needed a blood sample to check my blood count. If it was too low, the chemo would have to wait.

Thirty minutes later, Gwen and I were led back to the chemotherapy infusion area. Apparently, all systems were a go. With Gwen by my side, I settled into one of the recliners as the nurse checked the peripherally inserted central catheter (PICC) line that had been left in my arm after the Whipple surgery to provide long-term IV access without the need for needles. Once the nurse attached a line to my PICC, she began a hydration IV. Making sure the body is well hydrated during chemotherapy is important to help prevent kidney toxicity. The hydration solution gave way to a combination of steroids, Benadryl, and an anti-nausea drug to help counter side effects. While metronomic dosing reduces side effects, it doesn't necessarily eliminate all of them. This proactive drug trio could, however, better my odds.

Finally, an hour and a half after I had walked into the IV bay, the chemo cocktail was introduced into my IV line. Over the next six hours, it would seep into my bloodstream on a search-and-destroy mission. As the chemotherapy attacked the cancer, Gwen propped open my laptop. If I was going to be stuck here for hours on end, I figured that I might as well be productive. Gwen played secretary, reading my e-mails and taking dictation until the drugs kicked in. I dozed off and on as the hours rolled by, periodically punctuated with a visit from a variety of doctors and nurses.

Once the last of the chemo drugs had been pumped into me, the nurse flushed the IV line with a sterile saline solution and gently removed it from the PICC line in my arm. The combination of the drugs and the hours of chemo left me a bit lethargic. As the nurse helped me up from the recliner, she flashed me a sympathetic smile and asked, "Same time next week?"

The Aftermath

That night, I couldn't sleep. The steroids they had given me hours earlier left me wide wake and restless. But the worst was yet to come. Whether it was the fact that I had a form of GI cancer or that I was simply sensitive, nausea hit the next day. I was actually surprised. I had hoped the low doses of chemo drugs wouldn't trigger digestive problems. But, considering the option of not being treated, I decided that a little nausea was something I could live with.

Fortunately, I had been sent home with anti-nausea medication. Water—lots of it—also seemed to help. If I hadn't known better, I would have thought that I was flushing the toxins right out of my body by drinking so much. I also discovered that fresh air, and avoiding strong smells, helped immensely. But just knowing that I was taking active steps to eradicate this evil within me was my greatest weapon against my post-chemo discomfort.

A Conversation with Ben Chue, MD

Dr. Chue has been a pioneer in the use of metronomic chemotherapy, which effectively fights tumors while drastically reducing the often-debilitating side effects of traditional chemotherapy. Long before other oncologists, he offered promising, leading-edge treatments, including Herceptin for early-stage aggressive breast cancers and targeted therapy with the smart drug Rituxan for aggressive lymphoma.

Dr. Chue has been board-certified in both internal medicine and medical oncology. A graduate of Yale University with a degree in molecular biophysics and biochemistry, his internal medicine residency was at the University of Washington. He received his doctorate at the University of California, San Francisco. He is a clinical instructor at the University of Washington School of Medicine and has worked at the Fred Hutchinson Cancer Research Center, the University of Washington Cancer Center, and Virginia Mason Medical Center as a fellow in oncology. Dr. Chue has extensive experience in hematology and bone marrow transplants as well. He has conducted research in immunology, molecular biology, nutrition, obesity, and cancer at Yale University, the University of California, San Francisco, the National Institutes of Health, Rockefeller University, and the Fred Hutchinson Cancer Research Center.

Q: What attracted you to metronomic dosing?

A: As I was finishing up my fellowship at the University of Washington and the Fred Hutchinson Cancer Center, I began to notice that standard chemotherapy often didn't yield good results, and the side effects were extremely harsh. At best, chemotherapy could extend a patient's life by mere months, often at the expense of their quality of life.

But one event made me wonder if "traditional" chemotherapy was really in the patient's best interest. I was treating a woman with an advanced case of colon cancer. Since the cancer was aggressive, I knew I needed to use the usual maximum tolerated dose—yet I wanted to minimize her side effects. I decided to use 5-fluorouracil. This particular drug had been standard for colon cancer for many years and is considered one of the best tolerated of all chemotherapy drugs. I believed that it was her best option. Yes, there were potential side effects—diarrhea, nausea, vomiting, mouth sores, a poor appetite, and low blood counts—but I was confident that, as the standard treatment, this was the right course of action. I was wrong. The patient developed severe nausea and vomiting that resulted in life-threatening dehydration. For some reason, she didn't seek out medical attention and died within days of her treatment. My first reaction was to question the efficacy and tolerability of chemotherapy, and the wisdom of using it at all. Was it really worth it? In my gut, I knew that there must be a better way.

It was during that time that I came across two small studies that detailed the promising results of frequent low-dose chemotherapy for lung cancer. According to the researchers, they were seeing good results in their patients who had been treated with these low doses. The patients also suffered few, if any, side effects. I was intrigued. I ran the numbers and realized that, even though the patients weren't getting bombarded with the standard maximum dose every two to three weeks, giving them much smaller amounts more frequently actually resulted in a higher cumulative dose—without the ill effects often seen during chemotherapy. Perhaps this was the answer I had been looking for.

I began offering a weekly low-dose alternative to my patients and used a variety of individualized chemotherapy drug protocols. While many readily jumped on board this new concept, my colleagues were doubtful. Some who relied on conventional drug protocols like they were recipes in a cookbook were even convinced that I was harming patients instead of helping them. Yet I was seeing some remarkable results.

By the time I joined Seattle Cancer Treatment and Wellness Center in 1998, I was convinced that this was the future of chemotherapy for many types of devastating cancers, including lung, colon, and stomach cancer. I found a welcoming home at the progressive cancer center and began integrating metronomic dosing with complementary care that included naturopathy and acupuncture. As word spread, we found ourselves with some of the worst cancer cases imaginable. Each of these patients was looking for an alternative, and metronomic dosing seemed to fit the bill. During the first few years, we saw some incredible results—football size tumors that shrank to nothing and patients with no hope who recovered completely. Many patients who had been told by other oncologists that they only had three to six months to live gained years after our treatment. Some are still alive five or 10 years after completing therapy.

Of course, not all of the patients finished the treatment. And, not all of them survived. But the results were clear. Metronomic dosing works.

Q: You also don't always follow typical chemotherapy protocols. When did you first start looking at using other types of chemotherapy drugs?

A: It started many years ago when I began offering Herceptin to women with HER-2/neu+ early-stage aggressive breast cancer. At the time, Herceptin was a drug that doctors used only when breast cancer recurred in these patients—which often occurred, leading eventually to their deaths. But I saw the potential of Herceptin, especially when combined with paclitaxel from the yew tree and the platinum derivative carboplatin, to treat these patients with early aggressive breast cancer. This could prevent their disease from recurring and might cure them once and for all of their disease. I found that this combination of Herceptin and metronomic chemotherapy dosing did indeed prevent recurrence of this very aggressive cancer. I also discovered that metronomic dosing allowed greater amounts of the chemotherapy drugs to be given overall while, in many cases, reducing the incidence of side effects. The use of Herceptin, along with standard or metronomic dosing of chemotherapy (such as with paclitaxel) has now become standard for these aggressive tumors.

Q: How do you decide whether to use metronomic dosing or different chemotherapy protocols in patients?

A: If a certain protocol—even a conventional one—works, it may be the best option for patients. For instance, we know that treating testicular cancer with traditional chemotherapy offers a 99 percent cure rate. Hodgkin's lymphoma's success rate is 80 percent. These are wonderful statistics and, since good medicine means doing what is best for the patient, I don't mess with success. However, if I am treating a devastating cancer, like lung or pancreatic cancer, that doesn't respond well to conventional "high-dose" chemotherapy, I offer a different approach. You need to use what is best for each individual patient.

Q: You've been called a maverick by some of your colleagues. What is the goal of these less-than-conventional protocols?

A: My goal is not to do things differently just for the sake of doing things differently. I always look at the risk versus the benefit and what is in the best interest of the patient. Sometimes that means using conventional methods, and other times it requires thinking outside of the box. Often what starts as a less-than-conventional protocol becomes the new standard. Using what works is what matters. In Mark's case, we needed to take a different approach that targeted both the pancreatic and small bowel cancers. The outcome for both of these cancers is poor at best when you rely solely on traditional chemotherapy at traditional doses. It can also be very hard on the patient. By using different chemotherapy choices—for instance, oxaliplatin, paclitaxel, leucovorin, and 5-fluorouracil instead of the traditional gemcitabine, we were able to attack both types of cancer. Although this approach wasn't the standard practice, it was in Mark's best interest. And by using metronomic dosing, we were able to lessen the adverse affects of the chemotherapy. I am convinced that this less-than-conventional approach is why Mark has survived for more than three years as opposed to the six to 12 month prognosis most pancreatic cancer patients receive.

Q: When you use combination chemotherapy, what are you hoping will happen inside the body?

A: Killing cancer cells is the ultimate goal, either directly or indirectly. As cancer cells grow, divide, and form tumors, they develop blood vessels that protect and nourish the tumor in a process known as angiogenesis. Cancer is an extremely smart disease. It surrounds itself with a network of blood vessels that deflect chemotherapy and the immune system away from the cancer. The chemotherapy drugs and cells of the immune system essentially get lost before they can attack the cancer cells. This is one reason high doses of chemotherapy are often needed to have any impact on cancer, and why just trying to stimulate the immune system might not be enough to kill the cancer.

Along with the benefits I have already mentioned, I have found that frequent, low-dose chemotherapy also appears to block angiogenesis so that more of the chemotherapy, and perhaps immune cells, can reach the tumor bed. Certain chemotherapy drugs like paclitaxel can also hinder blood vessel formation by preventing endothelial cells—the cells that line blood vessels—from sticking together. Preventing this cell-to-cell adhesion stops the formation of new blood vessels that feed the tumor.

There are also other drugs, like interferon and thalidomide, that have anti-angiogenesis properties. Both of these drugs are sometimes used as treatment for various types of cancer. Oddly, this very same mechanism of preventing the growth of new blood vessels is precisely why thalidomide caused birth defects when it was given to expectant mothers in the early 1960s to ease morning sickness.

Q: Your chemo regimens often don't follow the standard protocols as far as the drug combinations you use. How does this impact the patient in terms of side effects?

A: It's very important to assess the side effects of each drug used and to make sure that the combination doesn't increase them. In other words, you don't want to use two chemotherapy drugs that have the same side effects if you don't have to. Doing so would simply increase the risk and severity of side effects. This can increase the possibility that the patient can't or won't complete treatment. At the same time, you try to find drugs that work synergistically to boost the efficacy of each drug used.

Q: What are the most serious side effects of chemotherapy? What strategies do you use to combat them?

A: While metronomic dosing doesn't automatically eliminate all side effects, it can reduce their severity. I have my patients who are bothered by side effects work with a naturopath and acupuncturist to address these problems naturally.

I've seen great success in reducing side effects and enhancing the efficacy of chemotherapy by adding specific herbs and nutrients. Peripheral neuropathy is a good example since the damage can be permanent if not addressed at the very beginning of a patient's treatment. In Mark's case, he was given two chemotherapy agents that carried risks of neuropathy—oxaliplatin and paclitaxel. To reduce the risk of neuropathy, he worked with naturopathic oncologist Dr. Paul Reilly, ND, LAc, FABNO, on a natural supplement regime that included glutamine, which decreases neuropathy that is triggered by paclitaxel, and IV glutathione for neuropathy caused by platinum derivatives.

Dr. Reilly and I had also found that a combination of calcium and magnesium reduced neuropathy symptoms, and Mark was taking both of these minerals. However, a preliminary study was released during his therapy suggesting that calcium and magnesium might actually decrease the effectiveness of platinum-based chemotherapy drugs like oxaliplatin. While I had never seen any evidence of this, Mark was given the choice to continue supplementation or suspend them. Mark chose to temporarily stop taking the two supplements. Fortunately, subsequent research showed that the scare over calcium and magnesium was totally unfounded. In fact, other studies have suggested that these two nutrients might even enhance the effectiveness of platinum-based drugs. But in the meantime, Mark's neuropathy became much, much worse. Although his neuropathy improved somewhat once he was back on the minerals, we might have prevented much of the nerve damage had Mark consistently taken them.

Q: You spent more than two hours talking with Mark and Gwen to make sure all of their questions were answered. What should patients ask their oncologist during their first appointment?

A: There are dozens of things that a patient wants to know about his or her illness, but these are the questions I consider most important during the initial appointment:

Is the diagnosis correct? All treatment is based on the diagnosis, so if the diagnosis is wrong, the treatment likely will be also. Obviously, this can be disastrous, yet it is surprising how often misdiagnosis occurs.

How bad is the cancer? It is important to be realistic. You need to know how advanced the cancer is and what the typical outcome is for the treatment your doctor is suggesting. On the other hand, just because the typical outcome may be a three- to six-month survival rate, don't ever assume that you are typical.

What are my chances of being "cured?" This can help a patient look for ways to better their odds.

What is your experience with this particular type of cancer? Each type of cancer has its own nuances so searching out someone with a track record of treating the specific type of cancer you have offers the greatest chance of successful treatment.

What are all my options? This will help you determine whether or not your doctor sticks strictly to textbook treatments or is willing to think outside of the box and look at non-standard options that are reasonable.

What is the timing of my treatment? Do you have time to get a second opinion? Can you postpone chemo, or should you get started right away?

What can I expect from here? Find out what the sequence of events will be and how many chemotherapy regimes the doctor anticipates to provide the best chance of eradicating the cancer and preventing recurrence.

How can I fight back? Ask the doctor what you, as a patient, can do to help yourself heal.

Q: How important is it to have a patient advocate?

A: Once a patient receives her diagnosis, the most important thing she can do is to find an advocate who will do everything in his power to put the needs of that patient first. This can be a friend or family member. However, it is ideal if you can find a doctor or medical professional who is practical, knowledgeable, and who does not let emotion cloud his decision-making. Doctors can often recommend other doctors who may be able to offer a different approach. They may also be aware of new therapies that are just coming to the forefront.

There are also advocacy groups that can help a patient who cannot find her own advocate. Many of these can be found either through national or community cancer organizations or on the Internet. (See Resources, page XX).

Q: How important is a patient's mental and emotional outlook to a successful outcome during cancer treatment?

A: A good attitude is critically important to a good outcome. If a patient has given up, the battle is already lost. But the patient's outlook isn't the only one that matters. The doctor also has to have the right attitude. Both doctor and patient have to believe that healing is possible so that they can get the best results from the treatment. Of course, you have to be realistic. But when both the doctor and the patient are willing to try a variety of approaches and not give up when standard therapies don't work, you can see some great successes.

Q: What do you see on the horizon for cancer treatment?

A: I am very excited about the future of cancer treatment. Based on what I have seen, I know that we can prolong survival and enhance the quality of life for patients with devastating cancers. I also feel like we are on the cusp of making cancer a chronic disease instead of a deadly one. This includes the "killer cancers" that have metastasized like lung cancer, colon cancer, and pancreatic cancer, which have traditionally had a very low survival rate.

I believe that we may even be able to cure many of these cancers in my lifetime. This may require new ways of thinking and novel therapies, but if these new ideas are based on science, there is an excellent chance that dying from cancer will become a thing of the past.

CHAPTER SIX

Complementing Chemo

Once you choose hope, anything's possible.

~ *Christopher Reeve*

MANY PEOPLE WHO UNDERGO METRONOMIC CHEMOTHERAPY experience reduced side effects. Standard chemotherapy, on the other hand, can trigger a number of side effects that are not readily controlled by the conventional prescription drugs I was familiar with. But thanks to Dr. Reilly, my side effects were, for the most part, tolerable. As one of an elite group of naturopaths who specialize in oncology, Dr. Reilly is genius at analyzing standard chemotherapy agents and utilizing naturopathic agents and combinations to not only minimize side effects but also enhance the efficacy of the chemotherapy.

I began working with Dr. Reilly before my first chemotherapy session. It was important to prepare my mind and body for what was to come. Many of the problems created by chemotherapy can be counteracted with a little bit of forethought and preparation. As I prepared for my therapy, I learned what would take place and the rationale behind Dr. Chue's chemotherapy choices. I also started to become familiar with Dr. Reilly's methods for preventing side effects. This was a huge stretch from my background in conventional pharmacology, but I was willing to take a leap of faith into the mysterious world of natural remedies. As I would learn in the coming weeks and months, it was a gamble that paid off with a wealth of benefits.

Soothing Side Effects Naturally

After just one chemotherapy session, I began to understand what people meant when they talked about the side effects of chemotherapy. While the fatigue and gastrointestinal problems were no picnic, the most maddening and painful side effect I experienced was peripheral neuropathy. It got to the point where I could not feel my feet and hands. Driving was no longer possible—not that I felt up to going out anyway. For a time, it seemed like chemotherapy and its side effects ruled my life.

Fortunately, Dr. Reilly was with me every step of the way with a variety of natural solutions to address both the side effects I could see and feel and the biological changes happening deep inside my body. Gradually, my laundry list of complaints eased to a level I could tolerate. I began to rediscover my interest in life as my energy levels increased— all thanks to a little help from Mother Nature.

Although I wasn't aware of it before I met Dr. Reilly, there is a global groundswell of research being done on the healing properties of vitamins, minerals, herbs, enzymes, and dietary supplements. Peer-reviewed lab experiments, animal studies, and even clinical trials are validating their ability to ease everyday maladies as well as prevent and even heal disease. I suppose I shouldn't have been surprised. After all, more than half of the prescription drugs I was familiar with are derived from chemicals first identified in plants. Aspirin is based on compounds in white willow bark. Codeine and morphine come from opium poppies. And paclitaxel, one of the drugs in my chemotherapy cocktail, comes from the Pacific yew tree.

There are so many natural remedies that can help tame the side effects of cancer treatment that it can leave a patient's head spinning. Here are some of herbs and nutrients Dr. Reilly recommended, as well as some other well-known natural medicines that can be used to soothe side effects. To be truly safe and effective, however, it's wise to work with a naturopath or certified herbalist well versed in integrative cancer therapies.

ACETYL-L-CARNITINE. Acetyl-l-carnitine is a molecule that occurs naturally in the brain, liver, and kidneys. Used as a supplement, preliminary research suggests that it may protect heart cells against the toxic side effects of the chemo drug doxorubicin without reducing the effectiveness of medication. There is also some evidence that acetyl-l-carnitine can improve peripheral neuropathy pain triggered by platinum-derived chemotherapy drugs like cisplatin and oxaliplatin.

ACTIVATED CHARCOAL. No, this isn't the kind of charcoal you'll find in your barbeque, although it does come from a similar source. Activated charcoal is derived from wood or other natural materials that have been heated in an airless environment. The resulting black powder can chemically attach itself to a variety of particles and gases in the digestive tract. Because of this, activated charcoal is very good at removing toxic substances—including excess chemotherapy drugs—from the digestive tract. Studies also show that it helps decrease the frequency and severity of diarrhea, especially diarrhea caused by the chemotherapy drug CPT-11.

AGED GARLIC EXTRACT. Animal and laboratory studies have shown that Aged Garlic Extract (AGE) enhances the activity of natural killer (NK) cells, macrophages, T-cells, phagocytes, lymphocytes, and cytokines. At least one clinical trial shows that it can do the same in people. The randomized, double-blind study, which was conducted at the Kyoto Prefectural University of Medicine in Japan, involved 55 patients with advanced liver, pancreatic, or colon cancer. The subjects were given either AGE or a placebo for six months. At the end of the study, the researchers found that, among those taking the AGE, both the number of NK cells and NK cell activity had increased significantly. Most AGE studies use Kyolic, a standardized odorless formulation of organic aged garlic.

ALOE VERA. Dr. Reilly suggested that I drink aloe vera juice while I was undergoing chemotherapy to soothe my gastrointestinal problems. A member of the lily family, aloe's healing powers have been touted since the fourth century B.C. It's no wonder. Aloe vera contains more than 70 essential oils, along with vitamins, minerals, proteins, enzymes, and amino acids. Aloe possesses remarkable anti-inflammatory properties that can calm irritated tissue in the GI tract. It also protects against opportunistic invaders like *E. coli* and *Candida* that can strike when immunity is low. There has been some debate over the safety of using aloe vera orally, however, so it is best to do so only under the supervision of a physician.

Used topically, some (but not all) studies show that aloe vera gel soothes burns and has well-documented wound-healing abilities. Two studies by the Chungbuk National University in Cheongju, South Korea, discovered that aloe vera gel contains tiny immunomodulators that prevent immune suppression in the skin when applied within the first 24 hours after a burn occurs. This can make it very useful if you are undergoing radiation therapy. Apply a liberal amount of pure aloe vera gel directly onto the area of affected skin to reduce inflammation and tissue damage.

ALPHA LIPOIC ACID. Known as the universal antioxidant, alpha lipoic acid has the ability to improve nerve function in cases of peripheral neuropathy. It also improves insulin action in the transport of sugar in the muscles. Since pancreatic cancer and type 2 diabetes often go hand in hand, this can be very beneficial.

CHROMIUM. Chromium functions as a key constituent of the glucose tolerance factor (GTF)—a compound that aids insulin in regulating blood sugar levels. It works closely with insulin to help the cells absorb glucose. Without chromium, the action of insulin is blocked and blood-sugar levels rise. Thanks to my former eating habits and my current cancer, I suffered from metabolic syndrome—a precursor of diabetes that consists of a constellation of symptoms, including high blood sugar levels, high cholesterol, elevated blood pressure, and abdominal obesity. Chromium helped keep the condition in check.

COENZYME Q10. Coenzyme Q10 is a nutrient that has gained enormous notoriety in recent years—and with good reason. Think of it as the Energizer Bunny of the cellular world. This novel enzyme is so important to cellular energy and good health that it's found in virtually every cell in your body. This is why CoQ10 is also called ubiquinone—it's ubiquitous in all cells. Without CoQ10, your body's cells, especially those in the heart, couldn't produce the energy they need to function. CoQ10 can also play a critical role if you are undergoing cancer treatment, especially if your chemotherapy includes anti-tumor antibiotics like doxorubicin. These antibiotics rob the heart of CoQ10, which leaves it vulnerable to damage. However, studies show that taking supplemental CoQ10 protects the heart from these toxic drugs. If that weren't reason enough to recommend it, preliminary data by researchers at Yonsei University College of Medicine in Seoul, South Korea, suggests that CoQ10 also discourages the formation of tiny blood vessels that feed cancer cells. It also reduces pain.

CURCUMIN. Found in the curry spice, turmeric, curcumin is multi-talented in the battle against cancer. Preclinical studies show that it inhibits the development of tumors in several types of cancer with a one-two punch. First, curcumin is able to interrupt the cycle of cancer cells. Second, it causes cancer cells to self-destruct by increasing p53 gene expression. P53 is a protein that suppresses tumor growth and helps maintain programmed cell death. A study by researchers at the University of Florida found that curcumin also interferes with the process that causes cancer cells to stick to each other, known as cell-cell adhesion pathway. What's more, curcumin discourages the formation of new blood vessels and boosts the body's own anticancer arsenal, including glutathione. There is also some speculation that curcumin can work synergistically with gemcitabine to positively impact advanced pancreatic cancer in some patients.

If that weren't enough, this remarkable spice inhibits the inflammatory response and oxidative stress. This means that it may be able to protect healthy cells against the damage that can occur during chemotherapy or radiation treatments.

While more research needs to be done on curcumin's anticancer activity, preliminary studies suggest that it is effective against pancreatic, prostate, breast, liver, stomach, colon, and skin cancer. It is extremely safe and can be used whether you are actively battling cancer or are looking to prevent the disease.

DEHYDROEPIANDROSTERONE (DHEA). One of the steroid hormones produced by the adrenal glands, DHEA is used for slowing or reversing weight loss and metabolic syndrome. Animal studies show that DHEA also increases immunity and cognitive function, while boosting strength, energy, and muscle mass. This can help prevent the muscle wasting that some cancer patients experience during chemotherapy.

This natural steroid may also have a direct impact on cancer cells. This was shown in one recent lab test that found DHEA inhibited the growth of cervical cancer cells. But, because DHEA can cause heart palpitations in some users when taken in high doses, it's advisable to only use this hormone under the supervision of your healthcare provider. Caution is also indicated in hormonally driven cancers like breast or prostate cancer, since DHEA can be converted into estrogen and testosterone.

DEGLYCYRRHIZINATED LICORICE (DGL). Long before Tums burst onto the scene, herbalists relied on plants to treat indigestion. The most effective and well-known choice was licorice. The problem with licorice, however, is that it contains a chemical called glycyrrhiza that can raise blood pressure. Fortunately, this dangerous compound can be removed and the resulting DGL is safe and effective. Popping a couple of DGL tablets before meals not only helps prevent heartburn, it's reputed to soothe and heal the esophageal tissue by decreasing inflammation and ulceration. Because it supports the stomach's healthy mucosal lining, DGL may also be helpful in treating ulcers of the duodenum, the first part of the small intestine. Make sure you use chewable tablets since DGL must mix with saliva to be activated.

FISH OIL. I've always been a big fan of fish. Of course, I preferred my fish battered and fried with a heaping side of French fries. Little did I know that other types of fish—fatty varieties like salmon, sardines, and herring—boast a special type of fat that not only helps guard against cancer but can help prevent many of the side effects of chemotherapy. It may even enhance chemo's effectiveness.

The oil from fatty fish contains two important types of omega-3 fatty acids: eicosapentaenoic acid (EPA) and docosahexaenoic acid (DHA). These fatty acids, especially EPA, enhance immunity and prevent severe weight loss and muscle wasting in cancer patients undergoing chemotherapy. A growing number of studies suggest that both DHA and EPA also enhance apoptosis, making fish oil an effective anticancer tool for the prevention of a variety of cancers, including cancers of the breast, colon, skin, pancreas, prostate, lung, and larynx. By implanting human tumors into immune-deficient mice, researchers have found that a diet high in fish oil can slow tumor growth. Plus, fish oil has been found to enhance certain chemotherapy drugs. Adding DHA to anthracycline-based chemotherapy can benefit breast cancer patients by making tumors more sensitive to treatment. And pairing supplemental fish oil with doxorubicin makes the drug more effective and increases survival.

FOLIC ACID. This B vitamin is necessary for normal cell replication and growth. It helps form the building blocks of DNA, the body's genetic information, and the building blocks of RNA, needed for protein synthesis in all cells. Because of this, rapidly growing tissues like red blood cells and immune cells have a high need for folic acid. Folic acid supplements also prevent mistakes from occurring during DNA replication and repair.

While this can provide some anticancer protection and help thwart infection if you are undergoing chemotherapy, there is some concern that high doses might actually contribute to the risk of certain cancers, especially prostate and breast cancer.

It's complicated. On one hand, a 2006 prospective study of 81,922 Swedish adults found that diets rich in folate reduced the risk of pancreatic cancer. A meta-analysis by New Zealand researchers has also concluded that supplementing with folic acid doesn't boost the risk of colorectal cancer. On the other hand, heart patients in Norway—where food is not enriched with folic acid—were more likely to die from cancer if they took folic acid and vitamin B12 supplements compared with those who did not take them. It could be that the devil is in the dose. Overloading the body with high levels of folic acid can prevent the body from metabolizing all of this B vitamin. This, in turn, is thought to reduce NK cell activity, which lowers the immune system's ability to defend against malignant cells. The bottom line is that, until more is known about folic acid's role in cancer prevention and treatment, your best option is to boost the amount of folate-rich foods in your diet. These include lentils, garbanzo beans, pinto beans, asparagus, spinach, and collard greens. If you do take supplemental folic acid, work with a doctor well-versed in nutritional supplements to find the proper dose.

GINGER. When chemotherapy leaves you nauseous, a hot cup of ginger tea can help settle your stomach. Researchers at the University of Southern California also discovered that this aromatic herb helps avert postoperative nausea and vomiting. While ginger is available in capsule form, a trial of 162 cancer patients undergoing chemotherapy found that ginger capsules did not alleviate nausea and vomiting. Opt instead for a cup of ginger tea or a glass of pure ginger ale like Reed's Natural Ginger Brew. You can also get some relief by sucking on a piece of ginger candy.

For the delayed nausea that often strikes a day or two after your chemotherapy session, try adding high-protein meals to your ginger. A clinical trial of 28 chemo patients revealed that those who drank a very high-protein drink and ate large amounts of ginger had significantly less post-chemo nausea and vomiting than the participants who consumed moderate amounts of protein and ginger.

GLUTAMINE. Glutamine is the most abundant amino acid in the body and is involved in more metabolic processes than any other amino acid. It serves as a source of fuel for cells lining the intestines. Without it, these cells waste away. It is also used by white blood cells and is important for immune function.

When it came to my own chemotherapy, I found that glutamine was one of the best ways to soothe my gastrointestinal side effects. I'm not alone. In one randomized crossover study, patients given glutamine intravenously experienced considerably less nausea, vomiting, and diarrhea than those who did not get the glutamine-spiked IV solution. It also helps reduce peripheral neuropathy in patients who, like me, are given a platinum derivative like oxaliplatin. It's so effective that it has become a key part of my therapy.

A SPOUSE'S PERSPECTIVE: Managing Multiple Supplements and Medications

With the incredible number of bottles and boxes to manage, I needed a system to organize Mark's many prescriptions and supplements. Complicating matters, some of the prescriptions are being actively taken, while others are held in reserve for future use. And, depending on Mark's needs, the supplements Dr. Reilly recommends often change monthly.

Anyone—whether patient or caregiver—faced with a myriad of pills and potions cluttering up the kitchen counter is faced with the same dilemma. Since it is critical that these medicines be taken properly, organization is of utmost importance. I don't know if mine is the most efficient system, but it works for us.

A section of our kitchen has become a mini-pharmacy. A large, deep drawer stores Mark's current supply of drugs and dietary supplements. These include vitamin C, CoQ-10, isoquercetin, Zyflamend, probiotic pearls, Neurochondria, Altace, Protonix, Lipitor, and antacids. This drawer also contains four oversized plastic pill trays that store the pills for the week. Two trays are needed for his morning dose, one tray is dedicated for the evening dose, and one holds his bedtime pills. I take inventory every weekend when I refill the trays so I can reorder his medications and supplements when needed.

Glutamine can be taken in supplemental form. You can also get a good dose of glutamine by adding whey protein to your shakes and smoothies. Whey protein—which is readily absorbed by the body—contains the highest concentrations of glutamine and branched chain amino acids found in nature. This promotes cellular health and efficient protein synthesis, both of which help to minimize the harmful effects of chemotherapy.

GLUTATHIONE. Glutathione is a small protein composed of three amino acids—cysteine, glutamic acid, and glycine—that naturally occurs in fresh fruits, vegetables, and lean meats. What makes glutathione so important to cancer patients is its ability to act like an antioxidant, an immune system booster, and a detoxifier. More specifically, it is involved in the synthesis and repair of DNA and the synthesis of protein. It also

---

Most people who are not facing a life threatening illness would probably consider this overwhelming enough, but it is only the tip of the iceberg in our house. A wall cabinet stores a supply of reserve supplements and over-the-counter drugs. And a specific spot in the refrigerator is set aside for the vial of Mark's interferon.

The centerpiece on our dining room table is a small tray of daily supplements, prescription drugs, and over-the-counter medications that don't fit neatly into the compartmentalized trays. They are easily accessible and include a canister of Sencha green tea, a bottle of fish oil capsules, vitamin D, maitake cell serum, aspirin, Pancrease, naproxen sodium, and Lactaid tablets.

Without a system like this, I would have been completely snowed under by the sheer number of pills Mark is required to take. Since Mark's health outcome and his ability to manage the side effects of chemotherapy are largely dependent of getting the timing and amount of his various medications and supplements right, coming up with a system was one of the most important things I could do to help him on his journey through cancer treatment.

— Gwen

metabolizes toxins and carcinogens, boosts the immune system, and prevents oxidative cell damage.

Some types of cancer have been linked to a glutathione deficiency, including oral, pharyngeal, colon, prostate, breast, and bladder cancer. But boosting your glutathione levels with supplements isn't very effective since it isn't well absorbed. When healthy subjects were given a single dose of up to 3,000 mg of glutathione, researchers found that it did not increase glutathione levels in the participants' blood. Fortunately, you can help your body make its own glutathione with vitamin C. Clinical trials show that blood glutathione levels rose nearly 50 percent in people taking 500 mg of vitamin C daily. In addition, several other nutrients can help increase glutathione levels, including N-acetylcysteine (NAC), alpha-lipoic acid, glutamine, and whey protein.

MEDICINAL MUSHROOMS. A variety of mushrooms—some culinary, some not—have powerful immune-boosting properties. Medicinal mushrooms are packed with nutrients like calcium, selenium, iron, vitamins C and D, and the B vitamins. Extracts are either water-based or alcohol-based and can contain one or more types of mushroom. Look for a standardized extract to make sure you're getting maximum immune-boosting power. Mushrooms are also a wonderful source of ergothioneine, an antioxidant thought to protect against cancer and cardiovascular disease.

- **CORDYCEPS.** This non-edible mushroom is often used in TCM to support male reproductive health. But it is far more valuable as a potent cancer fighter because of its ability to scavenge free radicals. A small study found that cordyceps also restored cellular immunological function and improved the quality of life in people with advanced cancer.

- **MAITAKE.** Since maitake increases natural killer cell function and reduces the symptoms of type 2 diabetes, it was a natural choice for my treatment plan. It's so effective against cancer that when investigators at Japan's Kobe Pharmaceutical University tested it in patients with advanced cancer, they found that maitake improved either the symptoms or the progression of the cancer in 58 percent of liver cancer patients, 69 percent of breast cancer patients, and 62 percent of lung cancer patients. They also found that immunity was enhanced when maitake was taken during chemotherapy.

- **REISHI.** One study in the *International Journal of Oncology* found that reishi can halt the proliferation of prostate cancer cells by causing them to commit suicide (apoptosis). Another recent study showed they help prevent breast cancer. Reishi is also a great tonic to boost overall immunity. A small 12-week trial involving 34 people with advanced-stage cancer found that those who were treated with 1,800 mg of reishi extract three times a day experienced a significant boost in immune function. Other studies suggest that this medicinal mushroom may also relieve chemo-induced nausea and vomiting.

- **SHIITAKE.** These tasty morsels contain lentinan, an active compound that stimulates the immune system. Since lentinan boosts intestinal immunity and fights infection throughout the body, it was a perfect fit for my situation.

MELATONIN. One of the primary side effects of chemotherapy is fatigue. And yet, even though you are bone tired, it's not unusual to experience insomnia. I found that I was literally sleepless in Seattle until I began taking melatonin. A hormone made in the pineal gland, melatonin is a popular supplement for jet lag and insomnia thanks to its ability to regulate the sleep-wake cycle. Often called the body's timekeeper, studies show that melatonin also helps alleviate stress and depression.

But melatonin's sleep and brain benefits might not be this hormone's only claim to fame. There is some speculation among scientists that it can improve immunity and encourage cancer cell death while protecting healthy cells. Melatonin has been used alone and combined with chemotherapy, radiation therapy, hormone therapy, or immunotherapy in a number of studies involving different types of cancer. These studies show that adding melatonin to conventional treatment can extend survival and improve the quality of life for patients with certain types of untreatable cancers such as advanced lung cancer and melanoma.

MULTIVITAMINS. In addition to specific nutrients designed to enhance your therapy and mitigate side effects, it's important to take a high quality multivitamin-multimineral complex. According to Centers for Disease Control and Prevention (CDC) surveys, only 11 percent of Americans meet the USDA's guidelines for eating five to nine servings of fresh fruit and vegetables daily. Because of this, nutrient shortfalls are dramatic. According to data gathered from 1999 to 2002 and compiled by the CDC, 93 percent of Americans don't get enough vitamin E, 56 percent don't get enough magnesium, 31 percent don't get enough vitamin C, and 12 percent don't get enough zinc. Another CDC survey indicated many people are low in vitamin K, calcium, and potassium, and many seniors lack the B vitamins. And deficiencies may be even more severe if you are having trouble eating during chemotherapy.

☙

Avoiding Post-Chemo Infections

Chemotherapy destroys cancer cells. It also kills healthy, infection-fighting white blood cells. This suppresses the immune system, making cancer patients more vulnerable to infection. Even a mildly depressed white cell count can reduce the body's ability to fight off foreign invaders.

Along with taking the immune-boosting supplements recommended by your healthcare provider, here are eight simple ways to boost your immunity and prevent post-chemotherapy infections.

* **WASH YOUR HANDS FREQUENTLY.** Be especially diligent about washing before and after eating, using the bathroom, and touching animals or children. Make sure you scrub your hands well. Doctors recommend washing for 20 seconds with soap and warm water. Time yourself by singing the "Happy Birthday" song twice through while you wash.

* **EAT A HEALTHY, BALANCED DIET.** Some chemotherapy patients experience a loss of appetite, nausea, and subsequent weight loss. In such cases, it's important to work with a dietitian to ensure a good diet and adequate caloric intake. Protein is especially important, because it is a basic building block used by your immune system to prevent and fight infections.

* **BE AWARE OF FOOD SAFETY ISSUES.** Careful food handling is important in avoiding illness. Cook meat and poultry thoroughly to kill any bacteria and other microorganisms that may be contained in raw foods, and be careful to avoid contaminating kitchen surfaces, cutting boards, and cooking utensils with raw meat juices. Additionally, steer clear of raw fish, seafood, meat, and eggs. All of these foods pose a high risk for causing illness.

A few years ago, studies began to surface from a variety of top research universities showing that multivitamins reduce the risk of chronic disease. Even the conservative *Journal of the American Medical Association* has stated that all adults should take a multivitamin every day. It's particularly important if you have cancer, since a multivitamin can help prevent nutritional deficiencies. And multivitamins

* **TAKE CARE OF YOUR TEETH AND GUMS.** Brush your teeth after meals and before bedtime, using an extra-soft toothbrush that won't hurt your gums. Floss gently, but talk to your doctor about whether flossing is the best way to protect your gums during chemotherapy treatment.

* **CULTIVATE HEALTHY SKIN.** Keep your skin hydrated and moisturized. Dry, cracked skin is more susceptible to infections. Furthermore, squeezing or scratching pimples can create open sores that would also place you at higher risk of infection. The same is true of biting or tearing at your cuticles.

* **KEEP YOUR BODY CLEAN.** Take a warm bath or shower every day and be sure to gently clean your rectal area after you use the bathroom. It's important to tell your physician if you develop hemorrhoids or dry, irritated skin.

* **STAY AWAY FROM PEOPLE WHO ARE SICK.** Because chemotherapy makes you more vulnerable to infections, it's important to avoid people who have colds, flu, chicken pox, measles, and other contagious illnesses. It's also a good idea to steer clear of people who have recently had a "live virus" vaccination, such as the chicken pox and polio vaccines.

* **AVOID ACCIDENTS AND INJURIES.** Wear gloves when gardening, be careful when handling sharp objects, and shave with an electric razor to prevent cuts. In the unfortunate event that you do get cut, scraped, or otherwise injured, be sure to clean the area with warm water and an antiseptic. The sooner you clean and cover the injury, the less risk there will be of infection.

contain micronutrients that you may not be getting from the foods you eat.

What should you look for when you are shopping for a multi? First, make sure that it contains all 12 essential vitamins (vitamins A, B6, B12, C, D, and E, as well as biotin, folic acid, niacin, pantothetic acid, riboflavin, and thiamin) at levels that meet or exceed the daily value set by the government. And, even though most of us just call it a multivitamin, it should contain minerals too, especially calcium, magnesium, manganese, potassium, selenium, and zinc.

PHOSPHATIDYLSERINE. Whether you call it "chemo brain," mental fog, or cognitive impairment, chemotherapy can definitely interfere with cognition and memory. Unfortunately, this is one side effect that can linger long after treatment stops. Phosphatidylserine, popularly known simply as PS, is an essential fatty acid that makes up part of every cell membrane in the body. It is most abundant in brain cells and allows nutrients and waste products to flow in and out of the cells.

A number of double-blind trials have validated the ability of supplemental plant-derived PS to improve memory, learning, concentration, word recall, and mood in middle-aged and elderly subjects suffering from age-related cognitive dysfunction. In one study, 15 elderly volunteers were given 100 mg of PS three times a day for 12 weeks. Researchers, who measured cognitive function at the beginning, middle, and end of the trial, found that 13 of the volunteers experienced significant improvement six weeks into the trial—an effect that was still going strong by the end of the study. A larger placebo-controlled study of nearly 500 elderly patients with cognitive impairment found that those taking a daily dose of PS had better cognitive skills after just six months compared to the participants taking a placebo. Most of the studies have used 300 mg of PS per day.

QUERCETIN. Like curcumin, quercetin protects healthy cells against the damaging effects of chemotherapy drugs and radiation. Which one should you use? That depends on which chemotherapy drugs you are taking. Dr. Reilly recommended that I take curcumin because I was also taking platinum derivatives as part of my chemo cocktail. However, studies show that quercetin can boost the effectiveness of other chemotherapy drugs, including antimetabolites (drugs that interfere with DNA and RNA growth), antitumor antibiotics, and microtubule- and

Be Supplement Smart

Buying high-quality supplements from a manufacturer you trust is only half the battle in making sure you are giving your body the nutrients it needs. Taking them properly can ensure that you're getting all the benefits they offer.

* Learn all you can about the supplement you are planning to take. Be particularly aware of any contraindications or drug interactions associated with the supplement.

* Store supplements in a cool, dry place. Check the expiration date periodically to make sure they are still potent.

* Timing is everything. Some supplements like calcium need to be taken in divided doses (i.e., two or more times a day) since your body can only absorb a limited amount at any one time.

* Unless otherwise instructed, always take your supplements with food. Taking them on an empty stomach can cause stomach upset and may prevent the absorption of fat-soluble nutrients. Taking certain supplements without food can also trigger unintended problems. Calcium, taken on an empty stomach, can increase the risk of kidney stones. Yet taking it with meals reduces risk, possibly by binding up the oxalates that contribute to kidney stone formation.

* Tell your doctor about every supplement you are taking. This is especially important if you are scheduled for surgery. Some supplements can interfere with anesthesia or cause excessive bleeding.

chromatin-inhibiting drugs that contribute to the process of apoptosis. Quercetin also sensitizes cancer cells so they are less likely to become resistant to drug therapy.

VITAMIN B1. Every cell of the body requires vitamin B1 to form adenosine triphosphate (ATP)—the fuel the body runs on. Nerve cells, in particular, require vitamin B1 in order to function normally. The problem is that four out of every six chemotherapy patients are deficient in this important B vitamin.

Often, a B1 deficiency can lead to peripheral neuropathy. But taking supplemental B1 may help reduce the pain and numbness. In one double-blind study of 24 patients with peripheral neuropathy, a high-dose B-complex supplement containing vitamin B1 significantly improved nerve conduction and reduced the pain and numbness.

VITAMIN B12. Vitamin B12 supports the insulation-like sheathing that protects the nerves and promotes the regeneration and growth of nerve cells. But a deficiency in this critical nutrient can make chemotherapy-induced peripheral neuropathy worse. People suffering from vitamin B12 neuropathy can experience weakness, twitching, pain, numbness, muscle cramps, burning, and tingling. Tongue soreness, appetite loss, and constipation have also been associated with vitamin B12 deficiency. While B12 supplements are readily available, most studies use B12 injections for maximum absorbability.

VITAMIN C. The best-known antioxidant is also one of the most powerful. Vitamin C is a water-soluble vitamin that the body cannot make on its own. But just because the body can't make it doesn't mean that it's not critical for good health. A potent antioxidant, vitamin C is necessary for the synthesis of collagen, an important structural component of blood vessels, tendons, ligaments, and bone. Vitamin C also plays an important role in the synthesis of the neurotransmitter norepinephrine, which is vital to brain function and mood. Plus it is required for the synthesis of carnitine, an amino-acid derivative that helps convert fat to energy.

When it comes to cancer, vitamin C has long been used to block free radicals that can damage cells and potentially lead to the disease. But fighting free radical damage isn't the only way vitamin C helps prevent cancer. It also neutralizes carcinogenic substances, enhances the immune system by increasing lymphocyte production, and stimulates collagen formation, which is essential for "walling off" tumors. According to one review of 46 studies by the National Cancer Institute, long-term intake of vitamin C was found to provide significant protection against cancers of the esophagus, larynx, mouth, stomach, colon, rectum, breast, cervix, lungs, and yes, pancreas.

But, while vitamin C is a nutrient most often used to prevent cancer, it may also help to treat it by encouraging apoptosis. New research suggests that large intravenous doses of vitamin C could reduce the size of cancerous tumors in people. In addition, if surgery is required, vitamin C may promote post-surgical healing by enhancing collagen formation. It may also increase tissue resistance to tumor spread.

Although these findings are preliminary, they could add to a growing amount of evidence that shows vitamin C can be an effective adjunct to cancer treatment when given through an IV. One animal study that appeared in the *Proceedings of the National Academy of Sciences* found that IV vitamin C produces hydrogen peroxide, which reduced cancerous ovarian, pancreatic, and brain tumors in mice by 43 to 51 percent.

Even though these results are very promising, not all of the experts agree that vitamin C should be used in cancer patients. Some oncologists cite a recent study that concluded that high doses of vitamin C actually diminishes the antitumor effects of common chemotherapy drugs. But there were two major problems with this conclusion. First, the study didn't use actual vitamin C (ascorbic acid). Instead, the researchers used an oxidized form of vitamin C (dehydroascorbic acid) that is not available as a dietary supplement for humans. The second problem? The mice used in the study were given toxic doses of dehydroascorbic acid. Fortunately, vitamin C has successfully been used in conjunction with chemotherapy for many years by alternative and complementary practitioners.

VITAMIN D. Known as "the sunshine vitamin," vitamin D has recently been found to be an effective nutrient for cancer protection, especially for hormone-related cancers. The problem is, many American are deficient in this important nutrient.

Vitamin D regulates cell growth and determines what a cell becomes, so a deficiency may allow cells to become cancerous rather than healthy. Based on this, researcher Cedric Garland and his team at the University of California, San Diego, examined 63 studies conducted between 1966 and 2004 that looked at possible links between a vitamin D deficiency and colon, breast, and ovarian cancer. They found that, out of 30 studies on colon cancer, 20 revealed a significant link between vitamin D and the risk of developing cancerous polyps and cancer mortality. Among 13 studies of breast cancer, nine reported a favorable association between adequate vitamin D levels and a lower risk of breast cancer. Five of the seven studies on ovarian cancer found that women who lived in colder climates with less sunlight or those with a lower vitamin D intake had a much higher risk of dying from ovarian cancer. The overall conclusion was that adequate amounts of vitamin D could slash these cancer rates by up to 50 percent. More recent studies support these findings.

What if you already suffer from cancer? Can vitamin D be used as part of a treatment protocol? Increasingly, the answer seems to be yes. Research suggests that vitamin D reduces the unregulated growth of cancer cells by promoting normal cell death. Test tube and animal studies also show that vitamin D prevents new cells from becoming cancerous. It even helps prevent cancer cells from spreading to other parts of the body and inhibits angiogenesis. While clinical trials need to be

---

✑

A Conversation with Paul Reilly, ND, LAc, FABNO

Dr. Paul Reilly is an incredible source of knowledge of naturopathic oncology. He is truly a genius when it comes to analyzing standard chemotherapy agents and utilizing naturopathic agents and combinations. His goal with these naturopathic agents is primarily to augment the efficacy of the prescription chemotherapy agents or utilize the naturopathic agent to minimize side effects.

One of the founding physicians at Seattle Cancer Treatment and Wellness Center, Dr. Reilly currently serves as National Director of Naturopathic Medicine for Cancer Treatment Centers of America (CTCA), overseeing naturopathic care at all of CTCA's hospitals. A board-certified naturopathic oncologist and a Fellow of the American Board of Naturopathic Oncology (FABNO), he is also a coauthor of *How to Prevent and Treat Cancer with Natural Medicine* (Riverhead Books, 2002), a practical guide for both cancer patients and those wishing to prevent cancer. In addition, Dr. Reilly was a contributor to the *Textbook of Natural Medicine*, writing the chapter on naturopathic oncology, and has published articles in the *Journal of Naturopathic Medicine, Townsend Letter for Doctors and Patients,* and *Health Store News.*

Along with his duties at CTCA, Dr. Reilly has served as a part-time faculty member at Bastyr University, where he graduated in 1985. He is licensed to practice naturopathic medicine in Washington and Oregon and also holds both national accreditation and state licensure as an acupuncturist.

Q: What led you to become trained in naturopathic oncology?

A: It basically grew organically out of a need I started seeing among the patients in my family practice. I realized how much

conducted to see if these effects translate to people, this could prove to be an incredibly valuable addition to the cancer treatment arsenal. One thing is clear, though: The current recommendations of 200 IU for people age 20 to 50 and 400 IU for those between 50 and 70 simply aren't high enough. Based on new evidence, most researchers now recommend a dose of 1,000 to 1,500 IU daily for maximum benefit, even for people without cancer.

---

people could do to improve their cancer outcomes and their quality of life utilizing complementary methods in addition to their conventional treatment.

Q: What makes naturopathic oncology different from conventional cancer treatment?

A: Naturopathic oncology focuses on the whole patient instead of just targeting the cancer. It looks at the underlying risk factors a patient may have, as well as the management of the patient's side effects. Because naturopathic oncology works in concert with traditional cancer treatment, it aims to amplify the benefits of conventional treatment at the same time it reduces side effects. It also addresses secondary prevention and overall wellness. Conventional treatment, on the other hand, takes a cytotoxic approach: Its sole goal is to kill the cancer with surgery, radiation, and/or chemotherapy. But, over the past few years, I have seen a gradual trend toward a more sophisticated and integrated approach as conventional oncologists slowly begin to take underlying factors into consideration and include more natural approaches during treatment.

Q: What should cancer patients look for when searching for a naturopath?

A: Qualified naturopathic physicians undergo rigorous training before they become licensed healthcare practitioners. Make sure the naturopath you see is a nationally accredited naturopath who has completed a four-year post-graduate degree, has taken the national board examination, and is licensed in the state in which she practices.

If your naturopath specializes in oncology, make sure she is board-certified by the American Board of Naturopathic Oncology (ABNO). Any naturopath with five years of experience who devotes 50 percent of her practice to cancer and is a member of the Oncology Association of Naturopathic Physicians is eligible to take this examination. Once she becomes board-certified, she will be a Fellow of the American Board of Naturopathic Oncology. This signifies that the doctor has advanced experience and knowledge in cancer care.

It's also important to find someone whose recommendations make sense for the average patient. You want recommendations that have proven science behind them and are not based solely on anecdotal reports. It's also wise to ask the doctor about her experience with cancer—particularly the type of cancer you have been diagnosed with. Cancer is a complex disease and treatment cannot be one-size-fits-all. The doctor should understand both complementary and conventional cancer care, as well as symptoms and side effects so that she can help guide you through your treatment.

Your naturopath should also be a good educator who can teach you about your disease and how you can participate in your own treatment. Lastly, it is critical that your naturopath is not only competent, but also compassionate. You want someone who will take that extra step, someone you can bond with and have confidence in.

Q: What questions should a patient ask during his first appointment with a naturopath?

A: After checking qualifications and making sure you feel comfortable with the naturopath, ask about typical treatment protocols. Does she recommend that you take a large number of supplements, do frequent juicing, or perform a colonic several times a day? Does she insist on adherence to an extremely strict diet? Are these recommendations you can live with, or do you need a protocol that is a bit more flexible and less demanding?

It is also extremely important that your naturopath communicates with your oncologist and other healthcare providers. I often send copies of my dictation notes and other information about my patients to their other doctors to ensure good communication about their progress. Is your naturopath willing to do this?

Q: What is the best way for a patient to approach his allopathic oncologists about using herbs and nutrients during chemotherapy?

A: I think it is important to select an oncologist who is comfortable with complementary medicine as an adjunct to your conventional treatment. Tell the oncologist that you will also be seeing a naturopath who specializes in cancer and chemotherapy or radiation. Ask if he or she is comfortable with that and will be willing to communicate and share information with your naturopath. If your oncologist refuses to do so, you may want to look for another one.

Q: Since supplements are widely available over-the-counter, what should patients be aware of if they are tempted to self-medicate—especially if they are undergoing chemotherapy or radiation?

A: While there are many dietary supplements that can be extremely useful in the fight against cancer, it is important to know that some nutrients can interfere with the effectiveness of radiation and chemotherapy. Even if a particular nutrient is cancer-specific, whether or not it is appropriate for your situation depends on a number of things including the type of treatment you are undergoing, your symptoms, and any underlying medical problems such as metabolic syndrome, hormonal balance, or immune deficiency. There are also specific supplements you should take before surgery and others that you should avoid because they cause excessive bleeding or other problems. What's more, the supplements you take depend on which chemotherapy drugs you are on. Only a trained naturopathic physician who has experience with cancer can match the most effective natural therapy with the specific conventional treatment a patient is undergoing.

Dosing should also be individualized. You can't use a standard dose and expect it to be effective for everyone. After all, the minimum dose listed on a supplement label is not a pharmacological dose. The appropriate dose depends on a multitude of factors—the size of the patient, the patient's metabolism, what other drugs and supplements he is taking, and the side effects that need to be managed. If you work with cancer a lot, you know these things.

When it comes to buying supplements, quality and potency are extremely critical. Up to 70 percent of time, supplements do not meet the label claims. This can make a big difference in a patient's chances for recovery. Another problem is that many of the cheaper brands of dietary supplements are adulterated with contaminants like heavy metals or fillers.

Q: Many conventional cancer specialists are not in favor of using antioxidants during chemo. What is their rationale?

A: Theoretically, the concern revolves around how chemotherapy and radiation work to kill cancer cells. Since both of these treatments generate free radicals that damage DNA, many doctors believe antioxidants (which fight free radicals) will interfere with the destruction of cancer cells. However, the published studies do not support this hypothesis. In fact, they show just the opposite. Antioxidants can actually improve the efficacy of treatment. Here's why: Both chemotherapy and radiation work in two stages. During the first stage, DNA is damaged. During the second stage, apoptosis (cell death) occurs. Antioxidants are key to the second stage. Without antioxidants, the efficacy of conventional treatment is actually reduced.

Another problem with this theory is that, if antioxidants were harmful, conventional oncologists would not recommend a diet rich in fruits and vegetables to their cancer patients. Fruits and vegetables are among the richest sources of antioxidants. Green tea is another dietary source of antioxidants. People in Japan routinely drink five to 10 cups of green tea each day, yet there are no reports that this polyphenol-rich beverage impedes chemotherapy.

⌀

Q: Are there any specific herbs that can help the body cope with the toxicity of chemotherapy?

A: There are, but again, you can't simply say that such-and-such herb can work in all situations. The most effective herb can vary depending on which chemotherapy drugs are being used. For instance, even though milk thistle is often the first herb considered for supporting the liver's ability to remove toxins, it isn't always indicated. Some studies do show that milk thistle reduces liver toxicity in children undergoing chemotherapy for acute lymphoblastic leukemia. However, the herb also activates cytochrome p450, which plays a key role in drug metabolism. This could potentially increase the level of chemotherapy drugs that are metabolized via this pathway, thus reducing the effective levels of the drug too quickly for maximum tumor-killing activity. This is just one example of why it is important to work with a naturopath who is knowledgeable in oncology.

There are, of course, exceptions. I tell all of my patients to drink plenty of water, which I consider the first level of cleansing. Combined with fiber-rich fruits and vegetables, water helps to flush toxins from the body. I also typically recommend that my patients take a multivitamin, as well as vitamin C and fish oil. Except for rare cases, these supplements are universally beneficial. For the majority of solid tumors, I usually rely on fish oil, melatonin, vitamin C, and mushroom extract.

Q: What do you see as the future of naturopathy in cancer care?

A: I see complementary medicine becoming a much bigger part of cancer care as time goes on. When we opened the Seattle Cancer Treatment and Wellness Center in 1997, what we did was considered quackery. Today, most mainstream doctors and cancer centers at least pay lip service to integrative medicine. In another 10 years, I believe that naturopathy will be fully integrated into every patient's care. But while conventional medicine catches up, integrative pioneers at CTCA and other progressive cancer centers aren't resting on their laurels. Instead they are conducting and compiling research on how complementary medicine improves patient outcomes. And that is what is most important.

The Antioxidant Controversy

Nothing ruffles the feathers of traditional oncologists more than the suggestion that antioxidants are a beneficial adjunct to chemotherapy. There is a belief among many oncologists that these free-radical fighters can render chemotherapy ineffective. They believe this because one of the ways chemotherapy works is by introducing free radicals into cancerous tissues to destroy them. They often cite a theoretical article that appeared several years ago claiming that antioxidants might undermine the effects of conventional chemotherapy and radiation. Accordingly, some doctors tell their patients to avoid antioxidant supplements during treatment. In fact, some doctors refuse to treat patients who are using antioxidant supplements. The problem is, there aren't any published studies to support their position. In fact, according to a systematic review in *Cancer Treatment Reviews*, antioxidants have the opposite effect and in fact enhance the effectiveness of chemotherapy and radiation, which can increase survival rates, tumor response, and the patient's ability to tolerate treatment.

In this review, scientists analyzed 19 studies involving 1,554 patients with a variety of cancers—many of them in the advanced stages. All of the studies showed better survival rates in those who took antioxidants than in those who didn't. People on antioxidants also responded better to their chemotherapy. When it came to side effects, the vast majority of patients in the antioxidant group also experienced the same or fewer problems like diarrhea, weight loss, nerve damage, and low blood counts.

This isn't the only study that shows antioxidants' benefit. Since the 1970s, 280 peer-reviewed *in vitro* and *in vivo* studies—including 50 human studies involving more than 8,500 patients—have consistently shown that antioxidants do not interfere with either chemotherapy and radiation. In 15 human studies, 3,738 patients who took over-the-counter antioxidants and other nutrients lived longer than expected. In one of these studies, researchers discovered that giving vitamin C and selenium simultaneously with the chemo drug Adriamycin increased the drug's effectiveness in mice. Preliminary research on humans also suggests that high doses of IV vitamin C (ascorbic acid) administered at 60 grams twice weekly can work synergistically with chemo to improve survival.

Other studies have found that glutathione; vitamins A, C, and E; ellagic acid; selenium; and beta carotene also enhance treatment. One common thread in most of the studies is that, with antioxidants, patients can typically avoid having to cut back on their chemotherapy dosing due to side effects. They are also less likely to need to interrupt scheduled treatments or abandon treatment altogether. A recent study of a group of colon cancer patients showed that those who completed their full schedules of chemotherapy had survival rates nearly double those of patients who abandoned their chemotherapy treatment prematurely.

According to Kenneth Conklin, MD, PhD, acupuncturist and anesthesiologist at the Ronald Reagan UCLA Medical Center in Los Angeles, "Nutritional factors may hold a key to enhancing the anticancer effects of chemotherapy and to reducing or preventing certain chemotherapy side effects." That's not to say that there's nothing to worry about when you combine supplemental nutrients or herbs with chemotherapy. Some may have undesirable consequences. For instance, an overabundance of supplemental copper can promote the growth of new blood vessels that fuel cancer. This may be of concern if you are also taking an angiogenesis inhibitor like Avastin. This is why it is best to take antioxidants and other dietary supplements under the supervision of a naturopath or other qualified practitioner of complementary or alternative medicine. It's also wise to keep your doctor and oncologist informed of any supplements you are taking.

CHAPTER SEVEN

A Healthier Way of Living

But he ate bacon every day!
~ *James Shigihara, written on the dry erase board*
in my hospital room.

FOOD HELPED GET ME INTO MY current predicament. It turns out that food can also help my body fight back against the cancer and keep me strong during treatment. The key is making smart food choices.

Studies have linked the typical Western diet to higher rates of cancer, and especially GI cancers. A diet filled with unhealthy fats, sugars, and empty calories also contributes to heart disease, stroke, diabetes, Alzheimer's disease, and other serious conditions. These ailments account for over half the deaths that occur each year in the United States.

According to CDC surveys, only 11 percent of Americans meet the USDA's guidelines for eating five to nine servings of fresh fruit and vegetables daily. Because of this, the dietary nutrient shortfalls are dramatic. According to data gathered from 1999 to 2002 and compiled by the CDC, 93 percent of Americans don't get enough vitamin E, 56 percent don't get enough magnesium, 31 percent don't get enough vitamin C, and 12 percent don't get enough zinc. Another CDC survey indicated that many people are low in vitamin K, calcium, and potassium, and many seniors lack the B vitamins. This is because many

Americans opt for fat-laden burgers over lean chicken or fish, chips over carrots and other vegetables, and sweets over fresh fruit. Sure these processed "foods" taste good, but they won't do a thing to promote good health. They simply provide calories, not quality nutrition.

I was as guilty as anyone. Without thinking, I routinely piled my plate with cheeseburgers, pizza, deep-fried chicken and fish, French fries, chips, cookies, pastries, and all manner of refined and processed goodies. Sure, I had high cholesterol, but popping a daily statin drug kept my lipids under control. Never in a million years did I stop to consider the impact all these tasty treats were having on my overall health.

Pop and Pancreatic Cancer

Studies suggest that drinking sugar-sweetened sodas can increase your risk of developing pancreatic cancer. One of the most recent was the Singapore Chinese Health Study, which involved more than 60,000 people. The 14-year study found that drinking two or more soft drinks a week elevated pancreatic cancer risk by an incredible 87 percent.

Since sugar—in the form of high fructose corn syrup—is the primary ingredient in soda, many scientists and nutritionists point to it as the cause of the increased risk. It's not far-fetched. In another large study, researchers looked at the diets of 180 women taking part in the Nurses' Health Study who had been diagnosed with pancreatic cancer. The investigators combed through 18 years of dietary records for each of these women, especially for carbohydrate intake and glycemic index. The glycemic index reflects the blood sugar response for each gram of a specific food. The researchers found a definite link between pancreatic cancer and a diet high in sugar, especially in the women who were overweight. These findings aren't really surprising, since tumor cells use more glucose than healthy cells do.

One 12-ounce can of soda contains about 130 calories, almost all of them from sugar. Regularly exposing your pancreas to this concentrated sugar-bomb can make it work overtime and eventually compromise its health. But choosing water or tea over sugary soft drinks can actually help protect your pancreas. It may be the easiest way yet to guard against pancreatic and other cancers.

But if I had looked at the emerging research, I would have realized that these foods were slowly killing me.

Was It Something I Ate?

Before I was diagnosed with cancer, my diet was a nutritional nightmare. Too much sugar, too much salt, and way too much fat, all of which undoubtedly contributed to my disease.

Of course, most of us already know that eating large amounts of refined sugar is unhealthy, but we often let our sweet-tooth get the better of us. Bad move! A high sugar intake causes a high glycemic load. Glycemic load is calculated using the glycemic index of the food and the total amount consumed. Since there is a link between glycemic load and the risk of diabetes, it makes sense to question whether it is also associated with a higher risk of pancreatic cancer risk. The evidence so far seems to indicate that it does. A study in the *Journal of the American Medical Association* concluded that having high blood sugar levels and diabetes almost doubled the risk of developing pancreatic cancer for men and more than doubled the risk of pancreatic cancer for women.

A study in the *British Journal of Cancer* also suggests that eating too much salt can increase the risk of stomach cancer. High levels of salt may cause the stomach lining to waste away. This condition, known as atrophic gastritis, can lead to stomach cancer. The study involved nearly 40,000 Japanese men and women between the ages of 40 and 59 years. The researchers measured the amount of salt people ate every day and followed them for an 11-year period. Their findings? Men who ate less than 6 grams of salt a day had a risk of one in 1,000 of developing stomach cancer. Men who ate 12 to 15 grams a day had a risk of one in 500. Women were a bit luckier. Those who ate less than 6 grams of salt a day had a risk of one in 2,000, with the risk rising to one in 1,300 for those who ate 12 to 15 grams a day. Now bear in mind that 15 grams of salt is only about three teaspoons. That much can be lurking in many of the processed foods that form the cornerstone of our diets. While the body needs some salt daily, most experts say that adding just 2.5 grams of salt to the diet each day is all it takes to meet our sodium needs.

Fat is another villain, particularly trans fat and saturated fat. Yes, the fat in that juicy burger or pepperoni pizza sure tastes good, but a steady diet of these grease bombs has been implicated in a variety of cancers, including breast, prostate, and colon cancer. When it comes to pancreatic cancer, a study by the Division of Cancer Epidemiology and Genetics at the National Cancer Institute recently made the connection after analyzing more than 500,000 people taking part in the National Institutes of Health–AARP Diet and Health Study. They found that those who ate large amounts of fat—particularly from red meat and dairy—had a 36 percent higher rate of developing pancreatic cancer compared with those who ate the least fat.

Red meat also has another strike against it if it's cooked improperly. Some studies have shown that frequently eating red meat cooked at high temperatures increases the risk of pancreatic cancer. Foods that are grilled, broiled, or fried form acrylamides, harmful chemicals that can damage the nervous system and cause gene mutations. A Swedish study found that acrylamides cause cancer in rats, and more studies are under way to confirm that they can do the same in humans.

Finally, there's processed meat. Sodium nitrates, the chemicals used in hot dogs, bacon, and other processed meats to help them look "fresh," form carcinogenic nitrosamines in the body. Nitrosamines are also triggered by food that are pickled, fried, or smoked, and things like beer, cheese, fish byproducts, and tobacco smoke.

A SAD Situation

The standard American diet (SAD) is based on what tastes good, not what's good for you. If you were to list the most important factors that contribute to the rise in cancer, heart disease, stroke, intestinal disorders, and diabetes, the typical American diet has them all. It's high in animal and manmade (trans) fats, sugar (often in the form of high fructose corn syrup), and processed foods. At the same time, it's low in fiber, complex carbohydrates, fruits, and vegetables.

A typical day for many Americans might start with a doughnut or muffin, coffee, and orange juice. Lunch would likely be a turkey sandwich with some chips or a hefty fast-food burger, a large order of French fries, and a super-sized soft drink. When your energy starts to wane, a mid-afternoon candy bar can prop you up until dinner, which often revolves around a big slab of meat accompanied by white rice or potatoes, a spoonful of corn or green beans, and a roll with margarine. And

A SPOUSE'S PERSPECTIVE: The Joy of Cooking

For Mark, cooking is a true passion. The joy in Mark's body language as he researches ingredients, plans meals, grocery shops, tweaks a recipe, and finally shares his tasty creations is evident. Our family chef enjoys every single start-to-finish step in preparing our meals.

While feasting on one of Mark's scrumptious masterpieces I once remarked that, had we lived in an earlier era or another culture, his zeal for cooking may not have been acceptable. Fortunately, that's not the case, since cooking is about as pleasurable for me as cleaning grout. My lack of enthusiasm has been repeatedly expressed in the form of bland taste and dull presentation. I am, however, quick to roll-up my shirt sleeves for most any home improvement project, whether indoors or out.

I do act as Mark's sous chef, slicing and dicing, washing dishes, or running to the supermarket for only the specific items on his grocery list. Cooking with Mark provides the opportunity to spend more blessed time together.

Since Mark's diagnosis, there has been upgrade in our family's diet. Our homemade meals had included white rice, chicken, red meat, seafood, fruits, and vegetables, but there was certainly room for improvement. Mark no longer cruises through the drive-thru when he is away from home and the ritual of Mark and the boys stopping for fast food after sporting events has been eliminated.

There have been sweeping changes for all of us. We've gone from guzzling a gallon of nonfat milk every day to drinking pitchers of filtered water. Teenage sons who once deboned pork chops now hunt for bones in their salmon fillets. The white rice that accompanied nearly every dinner has been replaced with a serving of brown rice. And leafy kale and spinach have become the familiar greens in salads, sandwiches, soups, and entrees. Surprisingly, James and Lane have made a seamless transition in accepting meals in this more nutritious game plan. They understand that it's not only for their father, but for their long-term health as well.

— Gwen

don't forget that bowl of ice cream for dessert. While this type of diet can fill you up, it's a prescription for a future health disaster. Yet, this is the way 88 percent of us eat every day.

What we eat has been linked to disease and premature death time and again. According to the CDC, 66 percent of us are overweight. What's even more alarming is that one-third of all Americans are classified as obese. The statistics for cancer aren't much better. The World Health Organization notes that what we eat accounts for about 30 percent of all cancers in countries that eat a Western diet. And the National Alliance for Nutrition and Activity—a legislative advocacy association made up of more than 300 health organizations—cites an unhealthy diet as the leading cause of early and avoidable death.

Even those who strive to eat a healthy diet can miss out on critical nutrients simply because of the way our food is grown and processed. Few farms today practice crop rotation, which allows the soil to build up the proper nutrients for another season's harvest. This means that the soil is missing many important nutrients, including chromium, zinc, and selenium, that are necessary for good health. The use of agricultural chemicals also reduces vitamin and mineral levels. One study found that application of pesticides to peaches and pears decreased vitamin C levels. What's more, our food loses nutrients during the time it's traveling from farm to table. Most of the fresh fruits and vegetables in our supermarkets are usually picked before they are ripe. The intention is for them to ripen during transport, but this does not allow for natural sun-ripening—and that results in reduced nutrients and flavor.

Processing also affects nutrient levels. While bread might have the reputation as the staff of life, don't try living on bread made with modern technology. To make that lovely loaf of white bread, millers use a high-heat process to remove the fibrous bran and germ from whole grains. Unfortunately, this fibrous material contains most of the plant's nutrition, including dietary fiber, B vitamins, and minerals like magnesium and zinc. Canned foods lose their vitamin and mineral potency primarily from the cooking and sterilization processes. Pasteurization is another potent destroyer of nutrients. To get the most nutrition from your diet—whether you have cancer or not—Dr. Reilly recommends eating foods as close to their natural state as possible.

The Importance of Organic

Luckily you don't need to settle for food that is filled with chemicals or has been manipulated beyond recognition. Today, grocery stores offer a growing variety of organic foods. But are they really healthier? Yes. Studies have shown that some organic foods are higher in antioxidants and powerful cancer-fighting nutrients such as conjugated linoleic acid. They're also safer because they are produced without dangerous pesticides or antibiotics. What's more, federal regulations forbid organic meat producers from using the risky practice of feeding animal byproducts to cattle. Certified organic products are the only foods available that have a government-backed guarantee that no chemicals, antibiotics, sewage sludge, or genetically modified organisms went into their growing or processing.

People who eat organic foods also reduce their pesticide intake by as much as 90 percent, according to a study from the University of Washington. Furthermore, research at the University of Colorado has found that certain strains of soil-borne bacteria found in organic fields not only stimulate the human immune system, but may also increase mood-boosting serotonin levels. Perhaps one of the prime advantages of organic food is that it is pure food, nothing more, nothing less. Forget hydrogenated fats, artificial colors and flavors, synthetic sweeteners, or preservatives. None of the additives lurking in processed and fast foods are permitted in organic foods.

Organic foods are also more nutritious than their conventional counterparts. Recent studies have found significantly higher levels of nutrients and antioxidants in organic produce. Analysis shows that organic foods have, on average, 27 percent more vitamin C, 29 percent more iron, and 14 percent more phosphorus. A study commissioned by the Canadian newspaper *Globe and Mail* and CTV news, found that today's conventionally grown potatoes contain 57 percent less vitamin C, 57 percent less iron, and 50 percent less riboflavin than they did 50 years ago. Modern industrial broccoli has 63 percent less calcium, 34 percent less iron, and less of seven other vital nutrients.

Not only are organic foods better for you, they are better for the planet. Fruits and vegetables grown using sustainable organic techniques promote biodiversity and protect air, soil, and groundwater. Instead of the brutal conditions that plague factory farms, organic meat, eggs, and dairy products come from animals that are treated humanely.

But how do you know you're really getting organic when you go to the grocery store? The USDA established national standards in 2002 to help consumers identify honest-to-goodness organic foods. Produce, meats, and packaged foods that meet the government's strict

---

How Much Is Enough?

In the 1970s, around 47 percent of Americans were overweight or obese; now 66 percent of us are. While increased portion sizes haven't been the sole contributor to our obesity epidemic, large quantities of cheap food have distorted our perceptions of what a typical meal is supposed to look like. But, with a little practice, you can reacquaint yourself with healthy portions.

If you are confused when reading a food label, try relating the portion size of a serving to everyday items. It is an easy way to visualize what a healthy portion size looks like.

* **Baseball**—a serving of vegetables or fruit should be about the size of a baseball.

* **A rounded handful**—about one-half cup cooked or raw veggies or cut fruit, a piece of fruit, or a half-cup of cooked rice or pasta would fit into your cupped hand.

* **Deck of cards**—a serving of meat, fish, or poultry.

* **Golf ball or large egg**—one quarter cup of dried fruit or nuts.

* **Tennis ball**—about one-half cup of ice cream.

* **Computer mouse**—about the size of a small baked potato.

* **Compact disc**—about the size of one serving of pancake or a small waffle.

* **Thumb tip**—about one teaspoon of peanut butter.

* **Six dice**—a serving of cheese.

It's also smart to get out a measuring cup or invest in a food scale and practice measuring some of your favorite foods onto a plate so that you can actually see how much (or how little!) a half cup or 3-ounce serving is. This will eventually help you "eyeball" a reasonable serving.

requirements are allowed to bear one of three "USDA Organic" certification seals. Products labeled "100 percent organic" must contain only organically produced ingredients. Those labeled simply "organic" must include at least 95 percent organically produced ingredients. And if the label says "made with organic ingredients," the product must be made of at least 70 percent organic ingredients. Even though organic foods are often more expensive than typical supermarket fare, the health and nutritional benefits—not to mention the peace of mind—you gain are well worth it.

Portion Distortion

It's not just what we eat that damages our health. It's also how much we eat. The recommended serving sizes of many of your favorite foods are often smaller—much smaller—than you think. The problem is that typical portion sizes for restaurant and packaged food has gradually nudged upward over the past 50 years. Muffins, sandwiches, and soft drinks have more than doubled in both size and calories. Twenty years ago, an 8-ounce cup of coffee with milk and sugar was a mere 45 calories. Today's 16-ounce mocha latte boasts 330 calories. My standby burger was just 250 calories when McDonald's first opened its doors in 1955. Now, however, the size of the typical fast-food burger has grown 500 percent and can top 1,000 calories. Add in large fries and a 64-ounce supersized soda, and lunch can easily weigh in at more than 2,000 calories—as much as the average person should be eating in an entire day! No wonder we are packing on the pounds and setting ourselves up for serious health problems, including cancer.

As food portions have grown over the years, so has the size of our plates. In the early 1990s, the standard size of a dinner plate increased from 10 to 12 inches. The size of our cups and bowls has also increased. Larger eating containers can influence how much you eat. A study published in the *American Journal of Preventive Medicine* found that when people were given larger bowls and spoons, they served themselves larger portions of ice cream and tended to eat the whole portion. Other studies have found similar results. Fortunately, you can easily downsize your portions by simply using smaller dishes. Instead of a dinner plate, try a nine-inch luncheon or even a seven-inch salad plate.

What to Eat When You Have Cancer

While good nutrition is important for everyone, it is critical if you have cancer. Not only do you need to make sure you are getting a sufficient number of calories and the right ratio of macronutrients, but you need to choose foods with cancer-fighting properties to help your body battle the disease. Fortifying your body with the right foods also helps you avoid malnutrition while you are undergoing chemotherapy. And according to Dr. Reilly, a healthy diet is even more important after you've finished chemo.

Dr. Reilly has developed a healthy eating plan specifically designed for cancer patients. It meets their particular nutritional needs before, during, and after chemotherapy and is bursting with healthy, nutrient-packed foods that play a direct role in the healing process. For a junk-food junkie like me, however, these foods were alien, and trading in my French fries for brown rice and broccoli certainly took some getting used to. It has taken all of my self control to stick with Dr. Reilly's eating recommendations. I must admit, given the choice between a double bacon cheeseburger and baked salmon with kale, my heart still leans toward the burger. Fortunately, my cancer, my doctors, and Gwen conspire to keep me on track.

Dr. Reilly's Anticancer Diet

Every healthy change you make moves you closer to long-term survival. That is Dr. Reilly's philosophy. He advises his patients to think of food as a biological response modifier—*this food moves me toward health and this other food does not.* You may not always choose the healthier option, but at least you know the risk and rewards when you make a choice. This gives you power over your health and puts you in charge.

Here are Dr. Reilly's recommendations—a cheat sheet, if you will—to help you make healthier choices.

PROTEIN. It's important, while going through cancer treatment, to increase your protein intake. This will help protect your body from weight loss and muscle breakdown. Chemotherapy and radiation damage healthy cells in addition to cancer cells. You need to have the protein building blocks—known as amino acids—available to make new cells. Adequate protein is also important for optimal immune function. High-quality, low-fat protein is best.

SMART PROTEIN PICKS	
ANIMAL SOURCES	**VEGETABLE SOURCES**
Cold-water fish like salmon, halibut, mackerel, sardines, and herring	Oats, barley, quinoa, amaranth, buckwheat, brown rice, millet
Free-range chicken and turkey	Soy, miso*
Organic eggs	Beans, lentils, legumes
Low-fat or nonfat yogurt	Nut and seed butters (e.g., almond, hemp)
Whey protein powder	Hummus
	Spirulina and soy protein powders*

* Avoid soy products (not soy foods) if you have an estrogen-dependent cancer like breast or prostate.

FATS AND OILS. Cook with extra virgin olive oil, extra virgin coconut oil, or organic grapeseed oil. It is also important to balance your ratio of omega-3 fatty acids and omega-6 fatty acids. Omega-3s are anti-inflammatory and possess many anticancer properties. They can be found in cold-water fish, certain nuts like walnuts, and flaxseeds. Omega-6s create inflammation and can be found in animal products as well as safflower, corn, and many other vegetable oils. The optimum ratio is 1:4 omega-3s to omega-6s.

SUGAR. Limit refined sugars since these can elevate your blood sugar levels. This has been shown to increase cancer growth. It's also important to be aware that white flour, honey, maple syrup, high fructose corn syrup, and highly processed foods are also sources of refined sugar. Unlike these refined carbohydrates, whole grains contain vitamins, minerals, and phytochemicals that contribute to good health.

Focus on foods with a low glycemic index. You can use a natural sugar substitute like stevia (an herb that is sweeter than sugar) or Lo Han Guo (a Chinese fruit extract). These sweet alternatives do not raise your blood sugar levels as rapidly as simple carbohydrates. However, on the day of chemotherapy, there may be a theoretical advantage to eating foods that increase your blood sugar, and therefore the metabolic activity of cancer cells. This makes them more susceptible to treatment. It also allows you to enjoy some of your favorite foods that you avoid during the rest of the week.

FIBER. Digestion plays a key role in your health. In fact, it is estimated that 80 percent of your immune system is in your gut. Adequate fiber contributes to a healthy digestive tract. Recommended daily fiber

---

Dr. Reilly's Master Smoothie Recipe

Smoothies are a practical way to get a protein and vitamin boost. Choose one or two items from each column and blend until smooth. Add water or ice to achieve desired consistency.

PROTEIN	VITAMINS/ MINERALS	FIBER	OMEGA-3S
Organic low-fat yogurt	Fruit	Oats	Fish oil
Organic Greek yogurt	Vegetables	Wheat germ	Ground flaxseed
Kefir	Kefir	Ground flaxseed	Nut butter
Protein powder	Spirulina	Fruits	
Spirulina	Chlorella		
Nut butter			
Bee pollen			
Soy or rice milk			

---

intake is 30 grams. Whole foods like fruit, vegetables, and whole grains are the best source of fiber. Cruciferous vegetables—broccoli, bok choy, Brussels sprouts, cabbage, cauliflower, and kale—are especially helpful for hormone-related cancers. Legumes and grains, especially lentils, beans, barley, oats, and ground flax seed meal have beneficial immune-stimulating properties. Just make sure to drink plenty of water when you are increasing your fiber intake. Try to drink at least half of your body weight in ounces of water (e.g., 70 ounces/day if you weigh 140 pounds). The combination of fiber and water will help you maintain daily bowel movements, which are crucial for removing toxins from your body.

ANTIOXIDANTS. The most well known cancer-fighting foods are fresh fruits and vegetables. Packed with powerful antioxidants, studies have shown that certain fruits and vegetables can protect against specific types of cancer. For instance, the lycopene in tomatoes may prevent prostate cancer as well as pancreatic cancer in men. Brussels sprouts and cauliflower benefit people with a genetic predisposition to lung cancer. Studies also suggest that berries and red grapes may have cancer-fighting properties.

Three recent studies have added even more evidence that, when it comes to cancer, antioxidant-rich foods can be the best medicine. Researchers in Milan, Italy, found that both onions and garlic help reduce the risk for colorectal, ovarian, prostate, breast, renal, esophageal, oral, and throat cancer. Another study at the Karolinska Institute in Sweden showed that eating lots of leafy greens and other carotenoid-rich foods can slash the risk of stomach cancer by half. These same foods may also reduce the odds of developing non-Hodgkin's lymphoma.

GREEN TEA. *Camellia sinensis*, the tea plant, is rich in anticancer flavonoids. Adding tea to your anticancer arsenal is a smart move. A recent U.S. Department of Agriculture study found that certain compounds in green tea called polyphenols kill human cancer cells. Drinking six to eight cups of green tea a day aids in cancer treatment at all stages, thwarting carcinogens and suppressing the growth and spread of tumors. Green tea is different than black tea because the fresh leaves are steamed to prevent oxidation. There are many types of green tea to choose from: green pearls, gunpowder, matcha, sencha, and jasmine. Try them all, then choose your favorites.

A practical way of drinking enough tea is to make a large batch in the morning and drink it throughout the day. If you are sensitive to caffeine, you can use decaffeinated tea.

ANTIOXIDANTS IN THE PRODUCE AISLE				
CAROTENES	**VITAMIN C**	**BIOFLAVO- NOIDS**	**VITAMIN E**	**SELENIUM/ ZINC**
Apricots	Blackberries	Apples	Avocado	Brazil nuts
Broccoli	Citrus fruits	Blueberries	Egg yolk	Cashews
Cantaloupe	Cruciferous	Cherries	Fish/shellfish	Cheese
Carrots	vegetables	Citrus fruits	Leafy greens	(low-fat)
Leafy greens	Guava	Green	Mango	Crab
Mango	Kiwi	pepper	Nuts	Eggs
Persimmons	Leafy greens	Green tea	Seeds	Garlic
Pumpkin	Mango	Herbs	Wheat germ	Halibut
Sweet	Melons	Onions	Whole grains	Oysters
potatoes	Papaya	White tea		Pumpkin
Tomatoes	Peppers			seeds
	Pineapple			Salmon
	Sweet			Scallops
	potatoes			Tuna
	Tomatoes			Whole grains

WATER. Drink at least six 8-ounce glasses of pure water each day. Water allows your cells to flush out waste products. Certain chemotherapies are irritating to the kidneys and it is crucial to stay hydrated. Drink spring or purified water as opposed to tap water since municipal and well water often contains contaminates that can harm health.

Cancer-Fighting Superfoods

Use this handy guide when planning your meals and making your grocery shopping list. Note: These guidelines are meant to be followed 80 to 90 percent of the time. Allowing for an occasional splurge will help you follow the plan on a long-term basis.

THE BEST FOODS			
Healthy foods that may inhibit cancer growth and are healthy overall			
FRUITS	**VEGETABLES**	**PROTEIN SOURCES**	**MISCELLANEOUS**
Açai Juice	Asparagus	Halibut	Almonds
Apples	Beans (all kinds)	Mackerel	Flax meal
Apricots	Beets	Nonfat yogurt	Green tea
Avocado	Beet greens	Salmon	Olive oil
Banana	Brussels sprouts	Sardines	Oolong tea
Blueberries	Cabbage	Soy milk	Spices & curries
Cherries	Carrots	Tofu	Spirulina
Cranberries	Cauliflower	Tuna	Walnuts
Guava	Celery	Whey protein powder	White tea
Kiwi	Dandelion greens		
Lemon	Garlic		
Lime	Greens		
Oranges	Kale		
Papaya	Lentils		
Pineapple	Onions		
Pomegranate	Parsley		
Prunes	Peas		
Pumpkin	Peppers		
Raspberries	Spinach		
Strawberries	Sweet potatoes		
Tangerine	Tomato		
	Vegetable juices		
	Winter squash		
	Zucchini		

GOOD FOODS

Basically healthy foods. Neutral action on cancer

FRUITS / VEGETABLES	GRAINS	PROTEIN SOURCES	MISCELLANEOUS
Corn	Brown Rice	Bison	Black pepper
Grapes	Grits	Calamari	Coffee
Honeydew	Millet	Clams/oysters	Dark chocolate
Plums	Oats	(cooked)	Peanuts
Potatoes	Quinoa	Duck	Pumpkin seeds
Watermelon	Rye	Eggs (organic)	
	Tortillas	Free-range chicken	
	Wheat bran	Free-range turkey	
	Wheat germ	Nonfat organic milk	
	Whole wheat	Shrimp	
		Swordfish	
		Wild game	

WORST FOODS

Unhealthy foods also suspected of helping cancer development or growth

FRUITS / VEGETABLES	MEAT AND DAIRY	GRAINS	MISCELLANEOUS
French fries	Bacon	Cake	Alcoholic beverages
Potato chips	Grilled meats	Cookies	Artificial coloring
	Hot dogs	Doughnuts	Artificial flavoring
	Ice cream	Sugary cereals	Aspartame
	Liverwurst		Beer
	Salami		Corn syrup
	Sausage		Cottonseed oil
			Deep-fried food
			Lard
			Maple syrup
			Margarine
			MSG
			Partially hydrogenated oils
			Saccharin
			Soft drinks
			Splenda
			Sugar

Staying Strong Through Chemotherapy

First and foremost, I needed to continue to keep my strength up, even if I didn't feel like eating. Even for someone who loved food as much as I did, eating turned into a daily struggle. After all, when you are nauseous, cramping, and running to the bathroom every half-hour, the last thing you want is lunch. As a result, I've lost 45 pounds since starting chemotherapy. I could have easily lost more weight had it not been for the supplements and helpful hints Dr. Reilly offered.

Along with my high-protein smoothies and increased fluid intake, I found the following tips helped me to get the nourishment I needed to handle my chemo treatments:

* If not provided, make sure to bring a light meal or snack to your chemotherapy sessions.

* Don't skip meals. If nausea or other gastrointestinal symptoms are a problem, tell your healthcare provider. There are a number of herbs and dietary supplements that can soothe stomach upset.

* Eat small, nutrient-dense mini-meals every two to three hours. Good options include a piece of fresh fruit along with a handful of walnuts or almonds, salmon salad on whole-grain crackers, or low-fat yogurt with fresh or frozen berries.

Chemotherapy can do strange things to your taste buds and your sense of smell. Favorite foods often don't taste or smell the same once you've started chemotherapy, and the flavor of sweet and bitter foods can seem intensified. You may have to use extra seasonings and spices to make food palatable.

Some people experience mouth sores during chemotherapy. If you are one of them, avoid foods like dry cereal and crackers. Focus on soft, moist foods like bananas, soups, puddings, smoothies, soft, starchy vegetables and legumes (like yams, squash, and lentils), and grains like quinoa and brown rice.

Falling Off the Wagon

As I've mentioned, there were times when adhering to my new anti-cancer diet was challenging. It still is. Sometimes it takes all of my self control to stick with my healthier eating plan. Fatty foods are my Achilles heel, and I still get cravings for pizza or burgers. And fried chicken—don't get me started! Avoiding sugar has been easier. I rarely ate sweets so desserts, juices, soda, and chocolate never held the same allure as greasy fast food. There is just something irresistible about devouring a juicy grilled hamburger and chasing it with a fistful of French fries.

Fortunately, Dr. Reilly is a merciful realist. He has told me that if I can adhere to his diet 90 percent of the time, it's acceptable to "cheat" on occasion. So if you see me at the drive-thru ordering a grease-filled burger with a side of fries, say a prayer for me and know that it is a rare event.

That said, I have been trying to increase the amount of healthy fish I eat because it is such a rich source of omega-3 fatty acids. I'm also eating an incredible number of vegetables each and every day, with a very heavy emphasis on kale, broccoli, carrots, celery, mushrooms, and green onions. Fresh fruit—something that was never a favorite in the past—also plays a crucial role in my diet. Antioxidant-rich blueberries have a prominent place in every breakfast for me.

But it's hard to exercise restraint and only opt for healthy foods 24/7. When I was recently hospitalized, the hospital had shifted its meal plan to a room-service type of system. Imagine that! I was in a shrine of health, and they allowed me access to a menu filled with the unhealthy foods I used to eat. I was just a phone call away from being able to order anything I wanted and in any amount. It was an all-you-can-eat buffet, delivered straight to my bed. Needless to say, I chalked that experience up to my 10 percent grace period.

Only saints are perfect all of the time—and I'm no saint. If, like me, you occasionally fall off the nutrition wagon, don't beat yourself up. It's OK to enjoy that occasional cheeseburger or piece of chocolate cake. Just make sure you don't make a habit of it. The 90/10 rule is designed to support the healing process in a way that most people can live with. *Bon appétit!*

Tips for Coping with Eating Problems During and After Chemotherapy

✳   Plan your major meal for the time of day when you are least likely to experience nausea and vomiting. Eating small, frequent meals and snacks through the day works well too.

✳   Let someone else prepare the food if cooking odors provoke nausea. Food served at room temperature or cold gives off less odor than hot food.

✳   If mouth sores are a problem, avoid salty, spicy, or acidic foods. Sucking on zinc lozenges may speed the healing of mouth sores.

✳   To overcome nausea, try chewing on ice chips or sucking on a ginger candy or sour lemon drop before eating. Sipping flat ginger ale or cola may also help.

✳   Rest for half an hour after eating, preferably in a sitting or upright position. Reclining or lying down may trigger reflux, nausea, and/ or vomiting.

✳   Pay extra attention to dental hygiene. Avoid full-strength products that can further irritate mouth sores. Try a baking soda paste and use a finger and a soft cloth to gently cleanse teeth. Rinse with a weak solution of hydrogen peroxide and baking soda.

✳   If dry mouth makes swallowing difficult, use a blender to liquefy foods or moisten them with low-fat milk, sauces, or gravies.

✳   If diarrhea is a problem, avoid fatty foods, raw fruits, whole-grain products, and other foods that can make it worse. Instead, eat bland, binding foods like rice, bananas, cooked apples, and dry toast.

CHAPTER EIGHT

The Advantages of Acupuncture

We've got magic to do.
~ Pippin

DR CHUE'S INTEGRATIVE APPROACH INCLUDES ACUPUNCTURE. When he first told me this would be part of my treatment plan, I was a bit wary. Even though this system of healing is more than 2,500 years old, it wasn't something I was familiar with. While there are studies on its efficacy, they aren't consistent. For a guy like me who is steeped in evidence-based conventional medicine, acupuncture was a real stretch.

Then there was the process itself. To be totally honest, I wasn't sure how I felt about dozens of tiny needles being inserted into my skin. Would it hurt? Was it safe? Yet, once I had survived my first session, I realized that I had nothing to worry about. In fact, the benefits I have received through acupuncture are truly astounding.

Of course, I didn't know this when I first met the man who would become my acupuncturist and an integral part of my cancer recovery. Darin J. Bunch, Dipl. Ac., MTCM, LAc, looks surprisingly young for one with so much knowledge of ancient healing techniques. Yet, his kind eyes and easy style made me feel instantly at ease. Like Dr. Chue and Dr. Reilly, he took plenty of time to explain the therapy and answer all of my questions. By the time I hopped up on the table for my first acupuncture session, I felt considerably more comfortable about becoming a human pincushion—even though I still didn't fully grasp the nuances of Qi, meridians, or how those little needles were going to make me feel better. In the end, I found that I didn't need to become an expert in acupuncture. It worked and that was what really mattered. Still, the general concepts of acupuncture and how it can help cancer patients are important to understand.

Acupuncture 101

Acupuncture is the most widely used type of TCM in America and is closely associated with Chinese meridian theory. According to this theory, there are 12 primary meridians, or channels, and eight additional meridians known as the Eight Extraordinary Vessels. Each of these meridians follows a particular directional course along the body. Qi, the inherent life force or energy in all living things, flows through these meridians and participates in regulating various bodily functions. Along the meridians are approximately 360 acupuncture points that serve as both a sign that something is wrong and as a location for acupuncture treatments. When the normal flow of energy over a meridian is obstructed (as a result of tissue injury or a tumor), pain or other symptoms result.

While most people think of acupuncture as the application of thin needles to these specific acupuncture points—a practice known as needling—there are actually several types of acupuncture. Other popular techniques include moxibustion and cupping. Moxibustion is a method in which a bundle of herbs—typically mugwort—is burned on top of an acupuncture needle or above the skin, warming it to alleviate symptoms. Although there have been no human studies of moxibustion's effect on cancer, a Taiwanese study did find that mice with tumors who had been treated with moxibustion lived longer than those who weren't treated.

Cupping involves burning herbs or other material in a glass, metal, or wooden cup. As the fire goes out, the cup is placed upside down over the Qi pathways, where it remains for five to 10 minutes. This promotes blood circulation and stimulates acupuncture points by creating a vacuum or negative pressure on the surface of the skin. This ancient acupuncture technique docs not have much in the way of peer-reviewed research to back it up. However, that may be changing as

Chinese scientists begin looking at the physiological evidence behind its effectiveness.

Acupressure, using fingers to apply pressure on acupuncture points, is also considered a form of acupuncture treatment. Like needling, acupressure opens the meridians and allows Qi to flow freely. And like traditional acupuncture, acupressure has been found to relieve the nausea and vomiting that can accompany chemotherapy. One study, conducted at the Institute for Health and Aging, University of California, San Francisco, found that women undergoing chemotherapy for breast cancer experienced considerably less nausea after acupressure treatments. The nausea they did experience was also less severe after treatment. Other studies show that acupressure can help ease nausea in patients undergoing radiation. Another benefit? It may help you sleep. According to Italian researchers, the use of acupressure can help cancer patients fall asleep and enhance the quality of sleep.

In addition to these classical acupuncture techniques, other techniques are sometimes used in cancer management. These include trigger-point acupuncture, laser acupuncture, and acupuncture point

---

Acupuncture is used to treat a wide variety of ailments. Its efficacy has become so well established that both the World Health Organization and the National Institutes of Health recognize its ability to treat dozens of common ailments, including the following.

Addiction	Diarrhea	Low back pain
Allergies	Dizziness	Menstrual cramps
Angina	Emphysema	Myofascial pain
Anxiety	Fatigue	Nausea
Anorexia	Fibromyalgia	Neuropathy
Arteriosclerosis	Food allergies	Osteoarthritis
Asthma	Gastritis	Rheumatoid arthritis
Bronchitis	Headache	Sinusitis
Carpal tunnel syndrome	Hypertension	Stress
Constipation	Indigestion	Stroke recovery
Dental pain	Insomnia	Tennis elbow
Depression	Intestinal weakness	Ulcer

injection. Acupuncture devices such as electroacupuncture (EA) machines and heat lamps can also be used to enhance the effects of classic acupuncture. Some techniques also focus on particular regions of the body: auricular (ear) acupuncture, scalp acupuncture, face acupuncture, hand acupuncture, nose acupuncture, and foot acupuncture. Of these, auricular acupuncture is the most commonly used.

Soothing Cancer's Side Effects

Practitioners of TCM believe that cancer occurs because the body's natural defenses have become weakened and compromised. While acupuncture is not used as a primary treatment for cancer itself, evidence suggests it can be a valuable therapy for cancer-related symptoms—

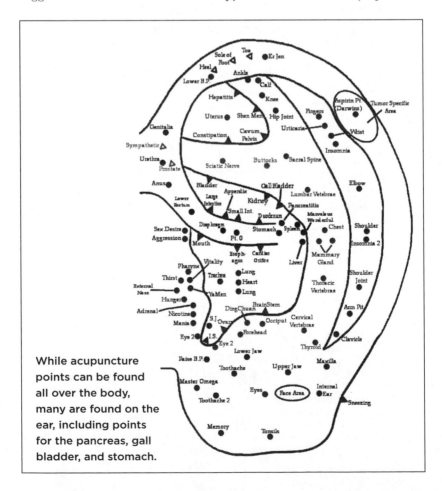

While acupuncture points can be found all over the body, many are found on the ear, including points for the pancreas, gall bladder, and stomach.

particularly the nausea and vomiting that often accompany chemotherapy treatment. One recent clinical trial conducted at China's National Pain Management and Research Center found that cancer patients undergoing traditional chemotherapy experienced significantly less nausea after receiving acupuncture than those who got sham acupuncture treatments. A recent meta-analysis of acupuncture trials by Johns Hopkins Sidney Kimmel Comprehensive Cancer Center also demonstrated that acupuncture significantly reduces chemotherapy-induced vomiting.

Other studies indicate that acupuncture reduces the pain commonly experienced by cancer patients. One trial pitted analgesics alone against

Acupuncture Angst?

When it comes to acupuncture, most patients want to know two things: Is it safe, and does it hurt? When done by a trained professional, acupuncture is extremely safe. The number of complications reported have been relatively few and are generally minor. The risk of infection is extremely low since acupuncturists in the United States use sterile, single use needles. Be aware, however, that bleeding and bruising problems are possible in patients who are also taking anticoagulants (blood thinners like warfarin). If bleeding is a concern, ask your acupuncturist to monitor your platelet count while you are undergoing treatment. People with cardiac pacemakers, infusion pumps, or other electrical devices should avoid electroacupuncture (acupuncture in which the needles are stimulated via small electrical currents).

As far as the experience itself, rest assured. Acupuncture is often less painful than getting a flu shot. The needles are extremely thin and sharp, and are inserted just deep enough into the skin to keep them from falling out. Once inserted, the acupuncturist may twirl the needles, gently tap them, or apply heat or a weak electrical current to enhance the effects of the therapy. You may feel tingling or a heavy sensation at the acupuncture point. The needles are usually left in place for anywhere from a few minutes to a half-hour depending on the objective. During this time, you may be surprised at how relaxed you feel. In fact, many patients—myself among them—even fall asleep during treatment!

a combination of pain-reducing drugs and acupuncture. After two weeks of treatment, the group receiving both the analgesics and the acupuncture reported considerably less pain than those receiving the drugs alone.

Then there is the fatigue that most patients experience after a chemo session. Everyday activities—talking on the telephone, shopping for groceries, even lifting a fork to eat—can become daunting tasks. Unless you've experienced it, it's hard to understand just how overwhelming it can be. When compared with the fatigue experienced by healthy people, cancer-related fatigue is more severe. It lasts longer and sleep just doesn't bring relief. There is little that can be done conventionally to ease this extreme fatigue, yet acupuncture seems to help—and it's not just a placebo effect. A randomized controlled trial by researchers at Britain's University of Manchester found that acupuncture really does ease the fatigue from chemotherapy. During the trial, 47 cancer patients received one of three types of treatment: acupuncture, acupressure, or sham acupressure. The acupuncture group received six 20-minute sessions over two weeks, while the patients in the two acupressure groups were taught to press either specific acupressure points or placebo points on the body. They were instructed to do this daily for two weeks on their own. At the end of the study, the participants all completed a Multidimensional Fatigue Inventory which revealed a 36 percent improvement in fatigue among those receiving acupuncture compared to just 19 percent in those performing acupressure and a mere 0.6 percent—hardly a blip on the radar—among those in the sham acupressure group.

Another important aspect of acupuncture during chemotherapy is that it can support the GI tract, including digestion and kidney function. This can help with the absorption and assimilation of food, nutritious beverages, and supplements that aid in the healing process. It also helps the body eliminate waste. Unfortunately, the importance of these biological systems is often overlooked during allopathic treatment.

Chemo Drugs and the Risk of Peripheral Neuropathy

Getting routine acupuncture treatments definitely helped control my chemo-induced side effects like nausea and fatigue. But perhaps the

COMMONLY USED CHEMOTHERAPY AGENTS ASSOCIATED WITH PERIPHERAL NEUROPATHY

Class of Chemotherapy Agent/ Specific Drugs	Incidence of Peripheral Neuropathy	Sensory Symptoms	Motor Symptoms
Taxane Class/ Paclitaxel Docetaxel Abraxane	60% 50% 71%	Mild to moderate numbness, tingling, burning/ stabbing pain of hands and feet are common and can become severe with increased doses. Reduced or absent Achilles tendon reflex.	Weakness of hand and foot muscles has been documented with high cumulative doses of paclitaxel and docetaxel.
Vinca Alkaloid Class/ Vincristine Vinorelbine	Not listed 25%	Mild to moderate numbness, tingling, burning/ stabbing pain of hands and feet are common and can become severe with increased doses. Reduced or absent Achilles tendon reflex.	Weakness of hand and foot muscles, decreased tendon reflexes, and foot drop have been noted with high doses.
Platinum Compounds/ Cisplatin Carboplatin Oxaliplatin	Not listed 4% 74%	Mild to moderate numbness and tingling of hands and feet can occur after prolonged (4-6 months) therapy and may develop 3-8 weeks after last dose. Symptoms can become severe with high cumulative doses. Reduced or absent Achilles tendon reflex.	Weakness is rare but can occur with high doses of cisplatin and oxaliplatin.

greatest benefit I received centered around improving my peripheral neuropathy. Peripheral neuropathy is a common side effect of chemotherapy, but it isn't something you hear about often. Some chemotherapy agents injure the peripheral nervous system, which is the system that transmits information between the central nervous system (the brain and spinal cord) and the rest of the body. As the nerves become damaged, patients can experience a sensation of pins and needles, pain, and numbness. For me, these sensations became so severe that I could no longer drive. Typing on my computer keyboard was all but impossible, and even holding a fork was a challenge.

While Darin gave me fair warning that chemotherapy-induced neuropathy is one of the most difficult side effects to treat, he implemented a variety of strategies—including acupuncture—to help repair at least some of the damage. Today, I can once again feel my extremities. I'm back in the driver's seat and have considerable use of my hands. Unfortunately, I will always suffer from some numbness and tingling. But the improvement I have experienced with acupuncture has been amazing.

Boosting Immunity

Acupuncture's effects go far beyond symptomatic. Careful attention is also given to strengthening and supporting the patient's natural defenses. Some researchers believe that cancer thrives when the immune system's defensive action can't or won't react properly. This lack of immune response may be due to age, toxic or viral damage, genetics, or even unique traits within the cancer cell itself that impact the immune response.

Impaired immunity may be why cancer spreads or even returns years after it has been defeated. The high incidence of metastases and cancer recurrence, even after surgery, chemotherapy, and radiation, attests that, although perhaps successful at wiping out the initial cancer, these treatments fail to restore the immune system's response to that of a non-cancer-prone individual.

Acupuncture works by stimulating specific portions of the autonomic nervous system, which, in turn, produces responses in the immune system. One Korean study found that acupuncture stimulation can cause a significant rise in blood levels of interferon, one of the immune system's messenger hormones. The effect lasts for several days and is much safer than other methods of boosting interferon. Several studies conducted in China on patients with malignant tumors also found that those who received acupuncture—whether or not they were also undergoing chemotherapy—had enhanced cellular immunity.

A Conversation with Darin Bunch, Dipl. Ac., MTCM, LAc

Darin Bunch has been studying and practicing acupuncture and Chinese medicine for more than a decade. I met Darin at the Seattle Cancer Treatment and Wellness Center when I went in for my first acupuncture treatment. I was pleasantly surprised. In addition to his wonderful bedside manner, Darin holds many advanced degrees. Along with a bachelor's degree in psychology from Seattle University, he has earned the degree of Master Traditional Chinese Medicine (MTCM) from the Northwest Institute of Acupuncture & Oriental Medicine. This is equivalent to earning master's degrees in acupuncture and Chinese herbal medicine. Darin is also certified as a Diplomat in Acupuncture by the National Certification Commission for Acupuncture and Oriental Medicine and is a member of the American Association of Oriental Medicine.

A lifelong student, Darin is always searching for ways to help his patients. He is one of only 18 candidates from around the world recently accepted into a clinical doctorate program at the Oregon College of Oriental Medicine. Upon completion of this two-year program, he will have earned his Doctorate of Acupuncture & Oriental Medicine—a distinction few practitioners hold.

Darin is constantly exploring the healing benefits of Asian modalities, including meditation, qigong, and tai chi. He also plays the role of teacher, sharing his wealth of knowledge with others. He has lectured at the University of Washington Medical School, Gilda's Club, Cancer Treatment Centers of America, and numerous public and professional conferences. Some of the topics of interest include managing cancer with acupuncture and traditional Chinese medicine, the integration of acupuncture and Chinese medicine in Western oncology, and the role of acupuncture and Chinese herbal medicine in healing and health. In addition, Darin has taught student interns from Bastyr University and the Northwest Institute of Acupuncture & Oriental Medicine. Needless to say, I was impressed during that first meeting. I still am.

Q: **What led you to focus on treating cancer patients?**

A: I began my journey in TCM when I was just 15 years old. A friend
of mine recommended an acupuncturist in Portland, Ore., to
help me with recurrent sinus headaches. I was curious about
the ancient healing practice of Chinese medicine—particularly
acupuncture and the alien use of needles to stimulate healing.
During that first appointment, I remember thinking that I must
have looked quite odd indeed. The needles that protruded
from either side of my nose reminded me of cat whiskers, while
the needle sticking out of my forehead made me think of a
unicorn's horn. Odd or not, I was delighted to discover that my
sinus headaches abated after only one treatment.

The headaches returned after I moved to San Diego when
I was 19. I again sought out acupuncture and Chinese medicine
at the Pacific College of Oriental Medicine's student clinic. But
when I arrived at the clinic for treatment, I did not realize that
I was going to be seen by a clinical supervisor and an entou-
rage of student interns. Bashful as I was, when they asked me
to remove my clothing and drape a blanket across my pelvic
area, I realized that this was not the clinic for me. Instead, I
turned to the Yellow Pages and made an appointment with an
experienced Chinese practitioner. After three treatments, I no
longer suffered from sinus headaches. I asked the doctor after
my final acupuncture treatment how one goes about becoming
a practitioner of Chinese medicine. He angrily replied, "You go
do something else—too many acupuncturists in California!" But
I was convinced that this was my true calling.

This belief was solidified in 1997 when my grandmother
was diagnosed with lung cancer. To my mind, her doctors
seemed to have a very linear view of treatment. They saw my
grandmother in terms of her disease without taking the person
into account. Don't get me wrong, her medical team was very
accurate with their diagnosis. And they really did try to offer
palliative care and treat her symptoms by removing the fluid
from her lungs. But they did nothing to support her immune
system, nothing to address the mind-body or psychoemotional
component to enhance the palliative care she received. There

was also no collaboration between the doctors—which meant there was little continuity in her care. Yet, this is what they were trained to do. These limitations, and the potential of a better way of treating people with life-threatening disease, are what led me to my eventual interest in helping those with cancer.

Q: Which acupuncture technique do you most rely on?

A: When working with cancer patients, I primarily rely on traditional acupuncture, Chinese herbal medicine, and heat therapy (far infrared magnetic heat lamps). I also use moxibustion, external liniments, and herbal plasters. Ear pellets or seeds, which are used to stimulate certain acupressure points in the ear, can also help ease anxiety, nausea (with or without vomiting), and various types of pain—including cancer-related pain.

Q: Do you use other modalities as well?

A: I often use what is known as plum-blossom or seven-star needling to activate certain acupoints. Plum-blossom is a technique in TCM, as well as a metaphor for a weapon used by several different Chinese martial arts. A plum blossom needle looks like a very small hammer with a group of needles on the head in the shape of a flower. I use this type of needle to tap gently along a meridian line to encourage the flow of energy along the channel. Plum blossom needling can often be employed to treat peripheral neuropathy.

Q: How does acupuncture help patients undergoing chemotherapy?

A: Acupuncture and TCM (including Chinese herbal medicine) can be of great benefit in reducing or managing the adverse reactions caused by chemotherapy regimens. Both of these modalities can help with fatigue, nausea and vomiting, pain, anxiety, depression, and low blood counts (red blood cells, white blood cells, and platelets).

Q: Can acupuncture help with neuropathic pain?

A: Chemotherapy-induced peripheral neuropathy can be stubborn to treat, but not impossible. I have seen good clinical results with neuropathy from diabetes, HIV, and AIDS. I've also found that polyneuropathies of unknown origin respond fairly quickly to acupuncture and Chinese medicine.

Q: Can you explain how acupuncture relieves pain in general?

A: There are several theories, but none fully explain the entire mechanism of how acupuncture works to ease pain. One theory suggests that acupuncture stimulates the body to produce narcotic-like substances called endorphins, which reduce pain. Other studies have found that pain-relieving substances called opioids may be released into the body during an acupuncture treatment. However, nothing to my knowledge has been definitively confirmed.

Q: Can acupuncture also relieve some of the stress cancer patients experience?

A: Absolutely! Acupuncture can help induce the parasympathetic nervous system response, which helps the body to relax.

Q: What is a typical acupuncture treatment like?

A: Because of the severity of a cancer diagnosis, it's not unusual for the first visit to take up to two hours. During that initial visit, I spend 45 minutes to one hour talking with the patient about appetite, digestion, bowel movements, urination, energy level, sleep, pain, psychoemotional status, and whether he feels hot, cold, or comfortable. I also ask him about his level of thirst and any particular cravings he may have. In addition, I take note of whether or not he has shortness of breath, heart palpitations, dizziness, or other specific symptoms. Once I have taken a complete history, I give the patient an opportunity to ask any questions he may have about acupuncture or TCM.

Next, a brief physical exam is performed, during which I look at the tongue and feel the radial artery pulses on each wrist. The patient is then instructed to lie on the table or sit in a chair or recliner. I begin treatment using hair-thin filiform or solid, sterile, surgical-grade stainless steel disposable acupuncture needles. Once the needles are in place, I gently manipulate them to obtain the desired therapeutic effect before leaving the patient to rest for 30 minutes or so. Often I will return to again gently manipulate the needles—up to three times during the course of treatment depending on an individual's sensitivity to the acupuncture needles.

Q: Do you think a patient's attitude toward acupuncture influences the success or failure of the treatments?

A: I believe that a good attitude can benefit the outcome of any treatment. However, I do not think that acupuncture and TCM are entirely dependent on a patient's attitude. I have treated many disbelievers who became my biggest advocates. These patients have been the best "marketing department" I could ever hope for.

Q: What is the biggest difference between Eastern and Western practices of treating disease?

A: In my experience with cancer, patients are not only suffering from a complex and often life-threatening illness, they are devastated at a psychoemotional level as well. While allopathic medicine can treat the disease, Chinese medicine can help offset the adverse reactions of the powerful Western treatments while focusing on the person as a whole rather than just the disease itself. I believe the integration of multidisciplinary healing modalities is often more beneficial in caring for a person diagnosed with cancer. I always see myself playing a key role in supporting and advocating for the integration of different healing modalities. Merging acupuncture and Chinese medicine with Western biomedicine is essential. Together, they are a powerful combination, each having its own strengths and weaknesses.

In the West, modern research—when paired with good research design—has demonstrated the powerful benefits of acupuncture and Chinese medicine. Gradually, Western medicine is becoming more accepting of the ancient healing methods of the East. Through education, scientific evaluation, and experiencing the validity of Chinese medicine, I believe many Western practitioners will begin to realize that we can better serve our patients by using the power of these combined modalities.

Q: Do you have any final thoughts?

A: I am so fortunate to be working at a cancer clinic that integrates Eastern and Western medicine. These two healing systems are like yin and yang. Together they create a dynamic duo for fighting cancer. But perhaps the most important components in healing are the patients themselves. I believe that patients should be encouraged to play an active role in their care. I may be teaching them about Chinese medicine, but my patients teach me every day.

CHAPTER NINE

The Mind-Body Connection

The secret of health for both mind and
body is not to mourn for the past,
worry about the future, or anticipate
troubles, but to live in the
present moment wisely and earnestly.
~ *The Buddha*

ANCER DOESN'T JUST AFFECT YOUR BODY. It also affects your mind. And what goes on in your mind—both intellectually and emotionally—influences what happens to your body. To put it simply, as we think, so we become. This is the premise behind many of the mind-body therapies used by a growing number of cancer patients.

I am so thankful that my medical team told me early on that stress reduction and other relaxation techniques could have a positive effect on the growth of my cancer. These exercises also help put things into perspective. I'm less likely to sweat the small stuff these days, opting instead to focus on the big-ticket goals like maintaining my health.

I also discovered that adding these less-than-conventional therapies to your cancer treatment gives you power. It helps put you in control. From the instant you receive a cancer diagnosis, a whirlwind of activity begins: constant tests, a series of doctor visits, surgery, chemo or radiation, and parade of pills. Among all this activity, it's not unusual to feel like a mere player in the drama that is unfolding in your life. The strategies in this chapter can help you cope.

Dealing with the Stress of Cancer

Let's face it: Life is stressful even when you are healthy. When you throw cancer into the mix, stress levels skyrocket—and chronic stress not only wreaks emotional havoc, it also impacts you on a physical level.

I am the kind of person who internalizes stress. Maybe this contributed to my cancer. Gwen, on the other hand, is an open book. She has to vent and release her stress and frustrations. She might be onto something, but I find that verbalizing the things that upset me isn't my style. Since my diagnosis, I have made a concerted effort to learn how to deal with the stress of cancer, work, and just everyday life through means more suited to my personality.

Music has been a wonderful escape for me. I particularly enjoy movie sound tracks because the composers create music which must be so skillfully constructed that a listener can remember key moments in a movie just by its melody. For example, John Williams' iconic score for the movie *The Empire Strikes Back* can stir visions of the menacing Darth Vader.

Music therapy has long been used to fight stress and manage pain. Studies show that it can enhance the quality of life in cancer patients, no matter what stage they are in. There is some evidence that, when used with conventional treatment, music therapy can help reduce pain and relieve chemotherapy-induced nausea and vomiting. Some studies have found that music therapy can even lower heart rate, blood pressure, and breathing rate. But you don't need to hire a music therapist or learn to play an instrument to reap these benefits. I've found that simply playing a favorite CD is often enough to transport me to another world and melt my stress away.

Another natural way I've found to ease stress is by cheering on our local sports teams. Many troubles have been forgotten—at least temporarily—as Gwen, the boys and I sit in Husky Stadium cheering on our team. Win or lose, I've realized that it's the time spent together that counts. I realize that this doesn't necessarily work for everyone. Some people can get extremely anxious and upset watching sports. If this sounds like you, look for a more relaxing form of stress relief.

How Stress Affects Your Body

To really understand the true scope of how stress can impact health, it's important to understand how worry, fear, and anxiety affect what's happening inside your body. When faced with danger—either real or perceived—people experience a complex chain of biological changes that instantly put us on alert. It begins in the hypothalamus, a tiny cluster of cells at the base of the brain that controls all automatic body functions. The hypothalamus triggers nerve cells to release nor-epinephrine, a hormone that tightens the muscles and sharpens the senses. At the same time, the adrenal glands release epinephrine, better known as adrenaline, which makes the heart pump faster and the lungs work harder to flood the body with oxygen. The adrenal glands also release the hormone cortisol, which helps the body convert sugar to energy. Once the threat has passed, the parasympathetic branch of the autonomic nervous system takes over, allowing the body to return to normal.

Unlike our ancestors who only had to deal with the occasional saber-toothed tiger or club-wielding enemy, we are often subjected to 50 or more stressors a day. Unfortunately, our bodies can't make the distinction between the life-threatening events like a fire and the frustration of being stuck in a traffic jam. As a result, stress-related healthcare costs have skyrocketed. In fact, it's estimated that 80 percent of all visits to the doctor are for stress-induced illnesses, including cardiovascular disease, diabetes, GI upset, skin problems, and neurological disorders, immune system dysfunction, and yes, cancer.

How can what goes on in your head have such a detrimental impact on your health? If you've ever gotten sick right after a stressful event, you've seen how stress can impact your immune system. Although the immune system is initially given a boost during the fight-or-flight response, persistent stress depletes nutrients like protein and B vitamins. Living in a world of wall-to-wall stress also results in immune-suppressing levels of the stress hormones epinephrine, norepinephrine, and cortisol.

Cortisol can also have a negative impact on the cardiovascular system. In a study of 18 healthy male doctors, researchers at the Humbolt University of Berlin, Germany, found that high cortisol levels can cause red blood cells to clump together. The blood becomes thick and sluggish, increasing the risk of hypertension, stroke, and heart attack.

Stress can also make a pre-existing medical condition worse. Diabetics are significantly affected by stress, since physical or psychological stressors can inhibit insulin production. People with seizure disorders such as epilepsy also find that stress can trigger an attack. In one retrospective study, Dutch scientists compared the seizure activity of 30 epileptic patients suddenly evacuated because of an impending flood to 30 patients living outside the evacuation area. What they found was that one-third of the evacuees experienced a significant increase in the frequency of their seizures compared to those who had not experienced the flood-related stress. People suffering from asthma are also more susceptible to attacks following a stressful event. According to researchers at the Kinki University School of Medicine in Osaka, Japan, stress causes the airway to become hypersensitive to histamine, resulting in wheezing and breathlessness.

Stress and Cancer

Chronic and acute stressors promote tumor growth. For the past decade, psychobiologist Shamgar Ben-Eliyahu, PhD, of Tel Aviv University in Israel, has been working on the link between stress, tumor development, and NK cells (or natural killer cells, a type of white blood cells). Of all the immune system cells, NK cells have shown the strongest links to preventing the spread of cancer.

It turns out that stress, including surgery and social confrontation, decreases NK-cell activity in rats for as little as an hour and as long as a day or two. What's more, these types of stressors cause a two- to five-fold increase in certain types of tumors and promote tumor metastasis. Stress may increase the risk of cancer on an even more fundamental level. Researchers at Ohio State University have found that stress impedes the cells' ability to repair DNA damage. Failure to repair DNA damage is one of the first stages of cancer development.

Other studies have gone as far as to show that women who experienced traumatic life events or losses in previous years have significantly higher rates of breast cancer. It makes sense, say a growing number of medical experts. If stress decreases the body's ability to fight disease, it loses the ability to kill cancer cells.

While cancer patients can't point to stress as the sole cause of their disease, it may be one of the many components in impeding their immune systems. The good news, however, is that, while we can't control our genes or family history, we can change how we respond to stress—and that could be one of the keys to preventing cancer and to helping control its spread.

Stress Less

No one expects you to take your cancer in stride. But there are a number of ways you can control how the stress of illness affects you, both mentally and physically. Here are some effective relaxation techniques to try.

AROMATHERAPY. Aromatherapy triggers changes in the brain that govern mood and emotions. Although aromatherapy should not be considered a miracle cure for serious emotional issues, it can—depending on the essential oil used—lift your spirits, calm you down, and boost your energy levels. Additionally, the proper use of essential oils may help you cope with the day-to-day challenges you face as a cancer patient.

Essential oils are composed of naturally occurring chemicals that work in synergy with one another. Because essential oils are volatile and evaporate quickly, their molecules are easily inhaled. The molecules then provide triggers to the areas of the brain that control our emotions. There is also evidence that certain scents can reduce pain, nausea, and depression.

If you want to try aromatherapy, make sure to use only pure essential oils. These highly concentrated oils are the volatile oils from herbs, barks, and flowers, which are processed via steam distillation or expression. Avoid products labeled as essence oils, perfume oils, or fragrance oils. Look for color variations and check the label for a statement warning against its undiluted use. This indicates that you are buying a pure, therapeutic-strength essential oil.

BIOFEEDBACK. Biofeedback is a treatment technique in which people are trained to improve their health by using signals from their own bodies. Using monitoring equipment, biofeedback is often aimed at changing habitual reactions to stress that can cause disease. Since many clinicians believe that some patients have forgotten how to relax, feedback of physical responses such as skin temperature and muscle tension provides information to help patients recognize a relaxed state.

Biofeedback can also help lessen pain. With proper training, you can reduce or eliminate symptoms and replace feelings of helplessness with a sense of control over your health. Biofeedback has also proven useful in retraining, reconditioning, and strengthening muscles after surgery, restoring loss of control due to pain or nerve damage (peripheral neuropathy), and overcoming urinary or bowel incontinence. Biofeedback can teach individuals, whether afflicted with cancer or not, techniques for living a healthier life overall.

During a biofeedback session, monitoring devices are used to amplify physical processes that can be hard to detect without help. This information is "fed back" in the form of a continuous signal (such as a tone or image readout). The person can then learn to adjust his or her thinking, emotional state, or other mental processes to change the signal and control his or her bodily functions. There are at least five different ways to measure bodily functions for biofeedback purposes:

* An electromyogram (EMG) measures the electrical activity of muscles. It is used in conventional medicine to diagnose a variety of nerve and muscle diseases and in biofeedback to help heal muscle injuries and relieve chronic pain and some types of incontinence.

* Thermal biofeedback provides information about skin temperature, which is a good indicator of blood flow. Several health problems such as migraine headaches, Raynaud's disease, anxiety, and high blood pressure are related to blood flow.

* Electrodermal activity (EDA) shows changes in perspiration rate, which is an indicator of anxiety.

ESSENTIAL OILS FOR EMOTIONAL WELL-BEING

Always dilute essential oils in a carrier oil like grapeseed, jojoba, or almond oil if you will be applying them to the skin. The typical ratio is 30 drops of essential oil to 1 ounce of carrier oil.

EMOTION	ESSENTIAL OIL	EMOTION	ESSENTIAL OIL
Anger	Bergamot, Jasmine, Neroli, Pettigrain, Rose, Ylang Ylang	Happiness/ Peace	Bergamot, Frankincense, Geranium, Grapefruit, Lemon, Orange, Rose
Anxiety	Bergamot, Clary Sage, Geranium, Lavender, Neroli, Patchouli, Sandalwood	Insecurity	Bergamot, Cedar, Jasmine, Sandalwood, Vetiver
Confidence	Bay Laurel, Cypress, Grapefruit, Jasmine, Orange, Rosemary	Irritability	Lavender, Mandarin, Neroli, Roman Chamomile
Depression	Bergamot, Clary Sage, Geranium, Grapefruit, Jasmine, Lavender, Lemon, Mandarin, Roman Chamomile, Rose, Sandalwood, Ylang Ylang	Loneliness	Bergamot, Clary Sage, Frankincense, Roman Chamomile, Rose
Fatigue	Basil, Clary Sage, Cypress, Ginger, Grapefruit, Jasmine, Lemon, Peppermint, Rosemary	Memory/ Concentration	Basil, Black Pepper, Cypress, Hyssop, Lemon, Peppermint, Rosemary
Fear	Bergamot, Cedar, Frankincense, Grapefruit, Jasmine, Lemon, Orange, Roman Chamomile	Panic	Frankincense, Helichrysum, Lavender, Neroli, Rose
Grief	Cypress, Frankincense, Neroli, Rose, Sandalwood, Vetiver	Stress	Bergamot, Clary Sage, Frankincense, Geranium, Grapefruit, Jasmine, Lavender, Mandarin, Patchouli, Rose

✳   Finger pulse measurements are used to reflect high blood pressure, heart beat irregularities, and anxiety.

✳   Breathing rate is also monitored. This measurement is used to treat asthma and hyperventilation, and to promote relaxation.

Biofeedback is often a matter of trial and error as patients learn to adjust their thinking. In time, they can connect changes in thought, breathing, posture, and muscle tension with changes in physical functions that are usually controlled unconsciously.

BREATHWORK. If you've ever heard the expression, "take a deep breath," you are already somewhat familiar with this relaxation technique. When we are stressed, our muscles tighten up and our breathing becomes shallow. As you breathe more lightly, you are participating in a vicious circle, because your body responds to your change in breathing with a fight-or-flight response, adding to your tension and stress. So the most basic thing you can do when you start to feel stressed is to stop and take some deep, slow breaths. There are many types of breathwork. Some, like qigong or yogic breathing, are best done under the guidance of an instructor. But just taking five or 10 deep breaths—and concentrating fully on each breath—can be tremendously helpful in soothing stressful moments.

HUMOR. Laughter is good for the soul, and recent studies indicate that using a little jocularity to manage stress can help reverse the damaging effects of stress hormones. Better yet, researchers at Indiana State University in Terre Haute have found that a good belly laugh boosts NK cell activity and increases overall immune function.

Besides keeping us physically and mentally balanced, humor can make us feel in charge of our lives, a feeling that's often missing in the face of a cancer diagnosis. While spontaneous laughter can be hard to come by when confronted by crisis, make an effort to look for the funny side of life. Create a humor bulletin board and tack up cartoons and jokes that make you chuckle. Regularly rent movies that leave you rolling on the floor. Collect silly things that make you laugh—children's toys, clown noses, funny hats—and play with them often. You might even try creating a "mirth-aid kit" full of things that tickle your funny bone for those times when stress gets the better of you.

MASSAGE. A host of mind-body benefits can be attributed to the age-old practice of therapeutic massage. According to the American Massage Therapists Association (AMTA), massage increases the body's supply of NK cells, which, in turn, boosts immunity and thwarts tumor growth. Massage can also increase circulation, reduce muscle tension, stimulate lymph drainage, control musculoskeletal pain, ease migraines, increase alertness and energy levels, and boost feelings of well-being.

There are a number of different types of massage. Eastern massage focuses on balancing the body's energy flow to produce good health. One type of Japanese massage uses choreographed movements that emphasize rhythm, pacing, precision, and form. Swedish massage approaches the body from an anatomical point of view and employs gliding, stroking, and friction to soothe the body. Aromatherapeutic massage combines the best of Swedish massage with aromatherapy to ease anxiety and fatigue. Whichever type of massage you choose, it's a good idea to find a certified therapist who is familiar with cancer patients. To get the most from massage therapy, plan on visiting your masseuse at least once a month, since the benefits aren't sustained or cumulative.

MEDITATION. As more and more people discover the benefits of meditation, the old counterculture image of navel-gazing gurus in a cloud of incense is being replaced by mainstream portraits of executives, athletes, and housewives, all engaging in this ancient practice. Learning to meditate not only helps put stress in perspective, it offers real health benefits. In one randomized study by the State University of New York, 16 adults with irritable bowel syndrome either participated in six weeks of meditation or simply had their condition monitored. By the end of the study, the symptoms of those in the meditation group had improved significantly compared to the control group. A year later, the researchers found that the meditators experienced even more relief as their practice continued.

Another recent study, conducted by the University of Wisconsin-Madison, found that meditation may have positive biological effects on the body's ability to fight infection and disease. The controlled 16-week study of 41 volunteers looked at the physiological effects of mindfulness meditation after all of the participants received a flu shot. During the study, the researchers measured levels of electrical activity in the frontal area of the brain and found that the meditation group's brains showed activity that indicated lower anxiety levels and a more positive emotional state. Better yet, although both groups had increased antibody levels in response to the vaccine, the meditation group had significantly larger increases after receiving the shots than the control group.

There are several different types of meditation, including mindfulness meditation, concentrative meditation, and transcendental meditation (TM). In mindfulness meditation, practitioners simply witness whatever goes through their minds without reacting or becoming involved with their thoughts and worries. Concentrative meditation focuses on something tangible—an image or a sound—in order to still the mind and allow a greater awareness to emerge. In both of these forms, the meditators become keenly aware of their reactions to stress, allowing them to gain a better sense of control over their lives.

Transcendental meditation is perhaps the most studied form of meditation. And, unlike mindfulness or concentrative meditation, TM is best taught by a trained professional. According to researchers at Reina Sofia Hospital in Cordoba, Spain, the regular practice of TM has a significant effect on the sympathetic nervous system. In their study, 19 practitioners of TM were compared with 16 volunteers who had never used any type of relaxation therapy. Throughout the study, the researchers measured the amounts of norepinephrine and epinephrine in the participants' blood and found that those practicing TM had consistently lower plasma levels of these stress hormones.

Meditation is especially well-suited to those battling cancer because it helps ease anxiety and promotes a sense of self-control. Studies of cancer patients show that meditation can change brainwaves, rejuvenate the central nervous system, and help people cope with their disease. A review of meditation and cancer by researchers at the University of Texas M.D. Anderson Cancer Center found that adopting a regular meditation practice can help improve cancer-related cognitive dysfunction—better known as "chemo brain." It also reduces stress, fatigue, nausea, and pain, and improves mood and sleep quality.

Although meditation appears simple in theory, it takes practice and patience to quiet the chatter in your brain. Since learning how to meditate can take some time, it's often best to take a class. Most communities offer both group and individual classes, which can be found online or in the local phone book. No matter which form of meditation you choose

5-Minute Relaxation Exercises to Try

Switch your thoughts to yourself and your breathing. Take a few deep breaths, exhaling slowly. Mentally scan your body. Notice areas that feel tense or cramped. Quickly loosen up these areas. Let go of as much tension as you can. Rotate your head in a smooth, circular motion once or twice. (Stop any movements that cause pain.) Roll your shoulders forward and backward several times. Let all of your muscles completely relax. Recall a pleasant thought for a few seconds. Take another deep breath and exhale slowly. You should feel more relaxed.

* **Close your eyes.** Breathe normally through your nose. As you exhale, silently say a short word such as "peace" or a short phrase like "I feel quiet." Continue for five minutes. If your mind wanders, gently remind yourself to think about your breathing and your chosen word or phrase. Let your breathing become slow and steady.

* **Pray.** Granted, not everyone has or wants a prayerful life, but for those who do, prayer can be a very helpful relaxation exercise. It can also help you feel that you are part of something else and that you are not alone.

* **Give yourself a mini-massage.** Try scheduling an appointment with a massage therapist who can teach you how to take care of your trouble spots while at work or home.

* **Apply heat.** If you have the option of a warm bath or shower, or simply have some warming gloves, socks, or heat packs, use the heat to help relax tight muscles.

* **Take a whiff of a soothing aromatherapeutic scent.** For an instant calming effect, keep a vial of lavender essential oil in your pocket, purse, or desk drawer so you can sniff any time you start to feel stressed-out.

to learn, find a quiet place and set aside 15 to 20 minutes once or twice a day to develop your practice.

TAI CHI. Although tai chi is a centuries-old offshoot of yoga, it departs from the still-life poses of yoga into the world of moving meditation. At the heart of the practice is the same Chinese concept of "chi" (qi) utilized in acupuncture. Often used as a relaxation technique, tai chi also improves concentration and balance.

Based on the movements of animals, tai chi is composed of slow dance-like steps and gestures. The weight of the body shifts continually from one foot to the other as the movements are performed in a series of circles, arcs, and spirals. The fluidity and grace of this form of exercise encourages relaxation and mental peace, as well as balance and flexibility. A qualified instructor is essential and classes are offered at many martial arts schools and health clubs.

VISUALIZATION. Many cancer patients use visualization, also known as guided imagery, to reduce stress and promote immune function. Visualization can trigger the release of brain chemicals that act as natural tranquilizers. This lowers blood pressure, heart rate, and anxiety levels. Researchers at Ohio State University in Columbus found that people with cancer who used visualization while receiving chemotherapy felt more relaxed, better prepared for their treatment, and more positive about their care than those who didn't use the technique.

Several studies suggest that visualization can also boost immunity. Danish researchers found increased NK cell activity among 10 college students who imagined that their immune systems were becoming very effective. At Michigan State University, researchers found that students could use guided imagery to improve the functioning of certain white cells called neutrophils, important immune cells in defense against bacterial and fungal infection. They could also decrease, but not increase, white cell counts. At one point in the study, a form of imagery intended to increase neutrophil count unexpectedly caused a drop instead. Subsequently, students were taught imagery explicitly intended to keep the neutrophil count steady, while increasing their effectiveness. Both of these goals were achieved.

Virtually anyone can successfully use visualization if they are willing to work at it. It's wise to practice your imagery for 15 to 20 minutes a day initially to ensure that you are learning to do it properly. As you become more skilled and comfortable with the technique, you will be able to do it for just a few minutes as needed throughout the day.

The most effective images are the ones that have some meaning to you. When battling tumors, people might imagine that their healthy cells are plump, juicy berries, while their cancerous cells are dried, shriveled pieces of fruit. They might picture their immune system as birds that fly in and pick up and carry away the raisin-like cancer cells, while the rest of the cells flourish. Another common image is that the immune system cells are like silver bullets coming in and annihilating the tumor cells.

YOGA. This ancient meditative art originated in India more than 5,000 years ago and takes its name from the ancient Sanskrit word for "union." In practice, yoga is simply a series of asanas, or poses, combined with a specific way of breathing that reduces stress, improves mental function, and exercises the body. And according to a study by doctors at King George's Medical College in Lucknow, India, yoga can also improve immune function. During the controlled trial of 60 healthy young men, half practiced yogic breathing on a regular basis, while the other half did not. Free radicals were measured in all of the volunteers at the beginning and end of the study. By the end of the trial, free radical levels were significantly lower in the yoga group, leading the researchers to conclude that yogic breathing not only helps relieve stress, but it can also improve a practitioner's antioxidant levels.

Since yoga can be adapted for any number of circumstances, you can take up a practice no matter what your age or fitness level. But, although there are a number of instructional books and video tapes on the market, yoga is best learned and practiced under the guidance of a qualified teacher. Fortunately, yoga centers are springing up across the country. You can also find classes at many health clubs, community centers, and colleges.

Exercise Your Options

While the activities I've just talked about can use the mind to impact the body, you can also use the body to affect the mind. In fact, exercising your body is one of the best adjuncts to an effective cancer treatment plan. Don't get me wrong—I didn't always subscribe to this belief. Prior to my diagnosis, I was anything but a workout warrior. I was an armchair athlete, wielding the remote control as I deftly flipped between whichever football or baseball games were on TV. For me, a bicep curl consisted of lifting a slice of pizza from my lap to my waiting mouth.

All that has changed. I now know that exercise is a key component of a healthy recovery. Exercise helps mobilize the body's own immunity. Physical activity can also help shift attention away from unpleasant or unhelpful thoughts and instead direct attention toward neutral or pleasant thoughts and activities. Diverting your attention, however, might be only part of the reason exercise is so effective at reducing anxiety. According to a recent study by the University of Southern Mississippi, 20-minute exercise stints throughout the day

The Benefits of Exercise

Thanks to cancer survivors like Lance Armstrong, a growing number of healthcare providers recognize exercise as a very important part of the cancer treatment plan. Little wonder, since exercise is credited with all the following benefits.

* Reduces chemotherapy-related fatigue
* Increases muscle strength
* Boosts energy
* Strengthens bones
* Helps reduce body fat
* Facilitates weight loss
* Improves insulin resistance
* Aids digestion and elimination
* Improves immune function
* Elevates mood
* Reduces stress
* Enhances mental function
* Improves sleep
* Increases self-esteem

can lower anxiety sensitivity. Not any type of exercise will do. The researchers found that aerobic exercise—walking, biking, or swimming—is most effective.

Due to my neuropathy, I have had to choose my exercise wisely to avoid falling. A primary activity for me is 30 minutes of walking daily. Since the weather here in Seattle often does not cooperate, much of my walking is done on a treadmill. It is easier on the body than pounding the pavement but still provides cardiovascular stimulation. Walking also helps me to maintain my independence. Combined with my other integrative treatments and the lifestyle changes I have made, I credit exercise with improving my health and fitness level to the point where I can work fulltime. For someone with stage 4 pancreatic cancer, that is remarkable indeed.

Your own exercise routine during cancer treatment will depend largely on how fit you were before you were diagnosed. Your doctor will be able to tell you if and how extensively you can exercise. If you do get the green light from your doctor, find a way to fit exercise into your life every day. Exercise, with adequate periods of rest built into your day, can boost your energy level, relieve stress, decrease anxiety and depression, and stimulate your appetite.

The benefits of exercise during and after chemotherapy and radiation treatment have been borne out in several studies. A recent review by researchers at the Swedish American Health System in Rockford, Illinois, concluded that a regular, committed exercise program resulted in less fatigue among cancer patients undergoing either chemotherapy or radiation. An early study conducted at my own school, the University of Washington, found that exercise also helps cancer patients maintain their weight and muscle strength during treatment. The 12-month randomized controlled trial involved 101 women who had undergone treatment for cancer. Each of the women followed either an aerobic exercise program or one that focused on resistance training. While both groups benefited, the aerobic exercisers saw significant improvements in their body composition (weight and lean muscle mass), aerobic capacity, and muscle strength. The researchers speculated that this, in turn, may also improve the participants' survival and quality of life. Other studies show that even people with advanced cancer can benefit from an exercise program.

How hard you exercise depends on your individual case and your doctor's recommendations. However, Danish researchers found that just having cancer and undergoing treatment doesn't automatically prevent a high-intensity workout. During the study, 269 cancer patients received either their regular conventional care or conventional care plus high-intensity cardiovascular and resistance training, relaxation and body awareness training, and massage for nine hours each week. After six weeks, the exercise group had less fatigue, more vitality, improved aerobic capacity and muscle strength, better physical function, and a greater sense of wellbeing than the control group.

Stick to It

Starting an exercise program is fairly easy. Sticking with it can be quite another matter. Every January, gyms and health clubs are filled with enthusiastic exercisers. But by April, many of these folks are nowhere to be seen. The goal, of course, is to make exercise a regular and enjoyable part of your daily life. Here are a few motivational tips to help keep you moving:

* **Find activities you enjoy.** After all, if you don't like exercising, you won't do it.

* **Get an exercise buddy.** Surrounding yourself with supportive people will keep you going.

* **Join an exercise class.** Just signing up for a class forces you to schedule it into your routine.

* **Try a trainer.** Professional trainers can help you remember why you started exercising in the first place. They can also make sure you have proper form.

* **Set exercise goals.** Tap into your competitive nature and see how long it takes to achieve your goals.

* **Keep a record of your activities.** Reward yourself at special milestones.

* **Vary your routine.** Doing the same thing every day becomes monotonous. Continually look for new ways to enjoy working out.

But, as beneficial as exercise can be, overdoing it can do more harm than good if you have been diagnosed with cancer. If you aren't used to exercising, start slowly. Try 15 minutes of walking every other day, gradually working your way up to at least 30 minutes daily. Over the course of a few weeks, you should notice a beneficial effect on your energy levels. If possible, increase the amount of time you walk to 60 minutes each day.

Adding resistance training like weight lifting to your exercise program can also help you feel better. Older cancer survivors showed greater strength and ability to perform daily tasks after resistance training, according to research presented at the 55th American College of Sports Medicine (ACSM) Annual Meeting in Indianapolis. Resistance training improves the muscles and nerve pathways that direct and control movement. It also increases bone density, strength, and general fitness, including enhanced function of the respiratory, cardiac, and metabolic systems. To prevent sore muscles and possible injury, it's wise to start slowly. Choose the lowest weight possible—two or five pounds—and start by doing 10 to 12 repetitions. Over the next few weeks, increase the amount of weight and the number of reps.

CHAPTER TEN

More Than Just Medicine

The Lord is my shepherd, I shall not want.
~ Psalm 23

L IKE A TSUNAMI THAT RISES UP from the sea with little warning, hearing those three words, "You have cancer," can send waves of emotion washing over you. Those words may terrify. They may trigger shock or deep sadness. There is no "standard" emotional response to cancer. Each person is different. For me, it felt like a house had been dropped on me. I was numb with disbelief, but I had to move forward.

Over the next few days, I experienced a profound sadness at the prospect of having my time with my family cut short. I worried about what would happen to my wife and children if I was gone. I was anxious about how I might respond to treatment. And I felt overwhelmed as I tried to mentally reorganize my life's priorities.

Not surprisingly, the nights that followed my diagnosis were the worst. Even if you live in a house full of people, 3 a.m. is a lonely time indeed. You are left with only your thoughts to keep you company. This is small comfort if all you can think about is the cancer.

Being diagnosed with cancer changes everything. Life is suddenly different in every way. Everything is about the cancer—your self image, your relationships, your plans for the future. The first thing you think about when you wake up in the morning is the cancer. It dictates how you will spend your day. Because the possibility of death is uppermost in your mind, every day now has a sense of urgency.

Many cancer patients say that the emotional rollercoaster after a cancer diagnosis is as bad as or even worse than the physical aspects of the disease itself. Whatever you felt when you were diagnosed will change over time. Some of these feelings will, as you would expect, be difficult. Anger, sadness, fear, and depression are all normal feelings as you start to cope with the fact that you have cancer. Oddly, however, so is relief—relief at finally knowing what's wrong, relief that treatment will soon begin to attack the cancer. You may also find an inner strength you didn't know you possessed. Comfort, in the form of family, friends, and even other cancer victims, can be very positive during treatment and recovery.

Whatever your initial reaction, give yourself some time to process your emotions. Not only is this important to your mental wellbeing, it can also influence the progression of your disease. A study of 32 women with recurrent breast cancer by researchers at George Washington University Medical Center found that those who bottled up their emotions died sooner than those who learned how to deal with their feelings.

Cancer, no matter what type or stage, is a big deal. There are no right emotions or wrong emotions. It's important to realize that it takes time to cope with this tsunami of feelings that suddenly wells up inside you as soon as you hear those three little words.

Dealing with Depression

Depression is quite possibly the most common feeling among cancer patients as they try to wrestle with their life-altering diagnosis. It's not uncommon to have trouble focusing on everyday tasks. You might even lose interest in basic activities like eating or grooming. Most people are able to work their way through this emotional funk on their own. However, if paralyzing depression lasts for more than a week or two, it's important to get help. Counseling can help you cope. Seek out a support group, learn how to express your emotions, educate yourself about your diagnosis, and take control of those lifestyle factors that can ease your journey.

What about antidepressants? There are many prescription and natural options that have documented effectiveness for depression. Depression is a very complex disease that requires close management with a medical professional. There is no one perfect antidepressant for all. Patients may respond in a different fashion if serotonin reuptake is inhibited alone or in combination with norepinephrine. Antidepressants are a dual-edged sword, though. They can have great efficacy, but patients need to be aware of potential side effects also. Just make sure to work with a physician, naturopath, or certified herbalist who is familiar with cancer before you take any type of antidepressant since they may interact with the drugs that are part of your treatment plan.

Anger Management

Anger is another common emotion for people living with cancer. It's OK and very normal to be angry in the wake of a cancer diagnosis. You might be angry that your body has been invaded by this awful disease. You may be angry that your life has been disrupted. You may be angry at how your disease has changed the relationships you have with family and friends. And you may be angry if the cancer has spread or recurred after a period of remission. All sorts of things can trigger anger when you have cancer and many of them are justified. But it's important to realize that anger can be either a negative or a positive force in your life.

You can channel your anger into a source of power to help you heal. It can also give you the strength and determination to fight the disease and complete treatment. However, if you bottle up your anger, it may contribute to anxious feelings and even lead to depression. Unresolved anger can also manifest itself through destructive behavior—some people abuse drugs or alcohol; some try to cope by pushing away the people they care about.

The best way to deal with anger is to identify it and find a way to express these feelings in a safe way. Here are some tips for coping with the anger that comes with cancer.

* **RECOGNIZE YOUR ANGER.** Surprisingly, it's not always apparent that you are harboring anger. Instead, you may find yourself acting out—yelling at your spouse or even a store clerk—without being aware that you are angry about something else.

* **DON'T TAKE YOUR ANGER OUT ON OTHERS.** It's easy to blow up at family and friends instead of focusing your anger on the cancer itself. This can drive away support just when you need it most.

* **DON'T HIDE BEHIND YOUR ANGER.** Anger may be just one of the emotions you are experiencing. Unfortunately, it can be used to mask these other painful feelings like loneliness, grief, or hopelessness. Dealing with all your emotions is important in the healing process.

* **DON'T LET YOUR ANGER BUILD UP.** The longer you let your anger simmer, the more destructive it can be when it is finally released.

Coping with Cancer

How you manage the physical and emotional aspects of cancer can have a great effect on the success of your treatment. It can also impact your well-being and the quality of your life day in and day out. The following coping strategies are adapted from *Everyone's Guide to Cancer Supportive Care* by Ernest Rosenbaum, MD.

* **Face the reality of your illness.** Patients who learn everything they can about their cancer and the pros and cons of various treatments tend to be better adjusted to their situation.

* **Maintain hope and optimism.** Patients who are hopeful and optimistic about the future course of events show a better adjustment to their illness than patients who are pessimistic. Some studies have also shown that optimism is associated with better medical outcomes.

* **Find proportion and balance.** Trying to be optimistic all of the time is an unrealistic goal. Yet letting anger, worry, and depression consume you is unhealthy. Try to balance your mental state to avoid these extremes.

* **Express your emotions.** Many studies show that people who talk about their feelings enjoy a better psychological adjustment to their illness than people who tend to suppress them. Find constructive ways to communicate your emotions.

* **Reach out for support.** Asking for help when you need it, whether it's emotional support or help with day-to-day tasks, is vitally important. Many patients also benefit from joining a support group where they can share concerns and information.

If you wait until your anger is at a critical level, you are likely to express it in an unhealthy way. Instead, deal with your anger as soon as you become aware of it. Vent to a trusted friend or counselor; release the full thrust of your anger while you are doing a physical activity like yard work or exercise; beat a pillow with your fists; or find a private space like the bathroom or your car, and yell and scream until your anger is exhausted.

* **Participate.** Don't be a bystander in your cancer care. Patients who participate in their treatment are more likely to have a positive state of mind and feel like they have at least some control over their situation. They are also more likely to pursue new or less conventional types of treatment that may benefit them.

* **Find a positive meaning.** While the diagnosis of cancer can be awful, it can also be an opportunity for positive change. This wake up call can be the trigger that moves you to re-evaluate your priorities or do the things you've always dreamed of.

* **Believe.** Having some type of spirituality or faith offers many benefits: a greater sense of peace, an inner strength, and an ability to cope. This translates to better psychological adjustment and quality of life.

* **Maintain self-esteem.** Cancer has always carried a stigma that can damage your self-esteem. The disease can also negatively impact your appearance, your physical abilities and activity level, your personal attributes, and your role within your family or social groups. Try not to let your cancer define you. Bolster your self-esteem by doing as many normal activities as possible.

* **Come to terms with your mortality.** While it's important to keep a positive attitude, it's also important to be realistic. Cancer increases the possibility of death. Unfortunately, there is very little support for patients trying to come to terms with this issue. However, the work of dealing with your own mortality can draw on your religious, spiritual, and philosophical beliefs about what is important in life and why. These beliefs can help you find meaning and a sense of peace.

The Healing Power of Attitude

Today, many people remark on my positive attitude, but don't be fooled: I was just as distraught as anyone would be after my diagnosis. However, I have learned how important it is to take the time needed to cope with the overwhelming emotions that a cancer diagnosis brings. I have also learned that how you process these emotions and the overall attitude you eventually adopt can be just as critical to the healing process as chemotherapy or radiation.

Dealing with your emotions can actually aid your journey through treatment and help take you into survival. The American Cancer Society reports that women in treatment who expressed their emotions, instead of suppressing those feelings, had stronger immune systems and better outcomes. A study done in 2008 at Utrecht University, in the Netherlands, found four themes that were common to patients who made a healthy adjustment to a severe diagnosis. According to the researchers, "patients should remain as active as is reasonably possible, acknowledge and express their emotions in a way that allows them to take control of their lives, engage in self-management, and try to focus on potential positive outcomes of their illness." These are all things I have tried to do in my own life.

Don't get me wrong, living with cancer is burdensome. However, there are positive aspects as well. For instance, cancer has given me a keen sense of focus. I now know that every day must be cherished. As one of my philosophical heroes, UCLA basketball coaching legend John Wooden, once said, "Make each day your masterpiece." I have taken this to heart. Every morning when I wake up, I try to set the tone for the day ahead with my attitude. Yes, circumstances and environments can affect me as the day goes on, but my attitude is the final determinant of whether or not the day will be a masterpiece.

Your overall perspective is also important. We've all heard the expression of the glass being half full or half empty. When you have a life threatening disease, it's like the glass has a crack. But instead of seeing the glass as flawed or broken, the optimist sees a glass with a unique design which can be filled up to the brim. The crack may prevent this, but the optimist overlooks the flaw and believes the attempt should be made. This type of optimistic attitude can have a huge bearing on many challenges. To believe the outcome will be positive is a gigantic initial step.

When faced with significant challenges, people often throw their hands up in submission because they have convinced themselves that there is no way the goal can be achieved. Their lack of optimism has doomed them to failure before the quest for the goal has even started.

In my role as a teacher and as a pharmaceutical consultant, I often speak to groups of students and colleagues about setting and meeting goals. While the people in the audience have different life experiences and come from different backgrounds, everyone can point to a time when they had to overcome an obstacle. While they may have had different methods for dealing with these individual challenges, they all found the inner strength to confront and overcome the problem. It's no different when you are faced with cancer.

But remember, it is you alone who is in control of your attitude. Do not be caught up in what can't be done; rather focus on what can be done. The ability to push forward through obstacles, disappointment, and failure is paramount. The true measure of a champion is the ability to rise from the canvas just one more time than you've been knocked down. Many consider a champion someone who does not fail, someone who escapes being knocked down. Yet, this is not realistic. There are dozens of examples throughout history of men and women who persevered in the face of failure, only to become successful. Abraham Lincoln, Harry Truman, Milton Hershey, and J.K. Rowling are just a few who come to mind.

To live life to the fullest, we need to avoid the fear of failure and attack life. I have made a solemn pledge to battle this disease no matter what challenges arise. For me the primary goal is to survive so I can spend more time with Gwen, James, and Lane.

Of course, there is a secondary goal as well, and it is one of the main motivations behind writing this book. When you are facing cancer, many of the things you hear come from doctors and other health professionals, well-meaning friends and family members, or so-called "experts." And much of the information you receive centers around conventional treatment. I felt it was important to offer another perspective from someone who knows the trials of living with cancer.

Keeping the Faith

Love, prayer, and a positive attitude have all been proven to aid the healing process. Personally, I believe that my faith allows me to have a

peace of mind that contributes to my overall well-being, both emotionally and physically. It also gives me perspective; it gives me hope. An
example of this peace of mind occurred the night of my eight-hour
Whipple surgery. Shortly before the surgery, Gwen and I met with the
hospital chaplain. After speaking with us for 15 minutes, he turned to

Most parents take on the role of teacher, passing down nuggets of
wisdom to their children. Yet there are times when our children can
teach us valuable lessons. Years before my own diagnosis, my son
James wrote an award winning essay about our neighbor, who was
an incredible cancer survivor. Little did I know that his report would
be a future key to my own recovery.

A LIFETIME OF COURAGE

The Olympic flame symbolizes the struggle for victory and spirit, so
it was fitting that on January 23, 2002, Tamara Stevens was one of
the runners who carried the Olympic torch for the Washington State
relay. For more than 30 years, she has willed herself to win against all
medical odds and revolutionize medicine in the process.

Two weeks before her 16th birthday in December of 1971, Tamara
went to see a doctor for a persistent cold. A blood test couldn't
detect any white blood cells so the doctors performed a bone
marrow aspiration out of her hip and still found nothing. Finally, a
bone marrow test from her sternum diagnosed Tamara with acute
myelogenous leukemia. Even though this type of leukemia had never
been treated successfully with chemotherapy before, the concerned
doctors still tried, but were unsuccessful.

Tamara's immune system was compromised and she was moved
to a restricted sterile room. She was unable to hang out with her
friends, which was a hardship for her. Tamara's weight had dete-
riorated to 88 pounds and she was five feet, seven inches tall! The
doctors said if Tamara could attain 99 pounds she could be dis-
charged. Well, this was a difficult challenge because, during her
chemotherapy, she had lost her sense of taste.

The desperate doctors tried a bone marrow transplant from
her brother. The procedure was a success, but later Tamara began
to reject her brother's bone marrow (graft versus host disease or
GVHD). The doctors had no other option but to give her a serum

Gwen and asked if I had already been sedated. I hadn't, yet I was at complete peace. No stress, no anxiety, just faith.

In this world there are many religions and beliefs. For myself, a belief in God helps me build perspective into my life. I know that my time on Earth is finite and I must do the best that I can with the gifts God

---

that had never been tried before to fight GVHD. It worked and it was a huge breakthrough in science! Previously, when patients rejected their transplanted organs (heart, bone marrow) they would die. Now, doctors had a way to treat GVHD.

Twenty-five years later, in May 1996, Tamara was diagnosed with stage 4 breast cancer, a result of radiation treatment for her leukemia. Many chemotherapy treatments have not halted the cancer from spreading to her liver and other parts of her body. It is a miracle that her body is ignoring it! Tamara believes that she is alive today because she has a positive attitude.

Also, she believes in God and the fact that she has too much to do—she can't die! She has set up a cancer information group for St. Madeleine Sophie, St. Margaret, and the Holy Cross Lutheran churches. It is a place where you can talk to people with the same type of cancer as you and be comforted. Tamara advises:

* Never believe the doctors when they tell you they can't do anything about your illness.
* Be with friends and forget your sickness.
* Have a regular day and believe that you will live.

The doctors told Tamara that she only had three months to live when she had leukemia, but she is still here 30 years later. When she had breast cancer, the doctors told her that she only had three weeks to live, but here she is, five-and-half years later.

Today, Tamara goes for 10 mile walks with friends as she practices for the next marathon. She is such an inspiration that, in the summer of 2002, Tamara received an award from another determined cancer survivor, Lance Armstrong.

I hope you can pass on Tamara's story to give others courage.

By James Shigihara
Neighbor of Tamara Stevens
November, 2002

has given me. There is a comfort in feeling that God has a role for me. No matter how difficult challenges become, I find solace in believing it is part of a bigger plan. To know God is to know peace of mind.

Prayers—my own and those of others—bring comfort. It is a powerful thing to know that others are praying for me as I travel this journey. My faith reminds me that I am not alone, that I am part of a larger whole. Disease often makes cancer patients feel cut off from community, even from themselves, and faith helps defy that sense of isolation.

Can prayer help you heal? I think it can—and there are studies suggesting that I'm right. An analysis of 43 studies on people with advanced cancer noted that those who reported spiritual well-being were able to cope more effectively with terminal illnesses and find meaning in their experience. Major themes of spiritual well-being included self-awareness, coping with stress, connectedness with others, faith, empowerment, confidence, and the ability to live with hope.

Other studies show that prayer may help reduce pain and speed recovery for a variety of diseases. In the late 1980s, a study in San Francisco found that heart patients who were prayed for by others appeared to have fewer complications. A larger study at a Kansas City hospital coronary care unit reported similar findings. Although the overall length of hospital stay and the time spent in the critical care unit did not differ between the groups, the group that had been prayed for had 11 percent fewer complications.

Personally, I gain internal strength from my faith. This is the foundation for the action I take when I attack problems that appear insurmountable. God has given us each unique gifts and I am convinced that faith allows us to believe it will be possible to overcome our challenges. I do not fear cancer. God has a plan for me and I am secure in knowing that I will be able to find a way to follow his teachings and make the world a better place.

CHAPTER ELEVEN

Dealing with Setbacks

*Resolve must be the firmer, spirit the bolder,
courage the greater, as our strength grows less.*
~ *Anonymous, The Battle of Maldon*

A S I WRITE THIS, I AM preparing to undergo chemo—again. Just when I think I have the upper hand, the cancer rears its ugly head to remind me that, when you have cancer, nothing is predictable.

Recently, lab tests showed that my tumor markers had gone up— not a good sign. But they weren't at stratospheric levels, so I was hopeful we could just keep a watchful eye on them or maybe just tweak my medication. After reviewing my test results, Dr. Chue and his Seattle Cancer Treatment and Wellness Center associate, Dr. James Cunningham agreed. Hoping that the rest of my oncology team would concur, I called my coauthor, Kim, to give her the good news. I was so hopeful—perhaps a little too hopeful.

This current round of chemo was preceded by an acute, and extremely painful, attack of pancreatitis on Easter Sunday. It struck just as we were finishing a wonderful family luncheon with Gwen's family in Seattle. As everyone chatted happily, I began feeling ill. Over the next 12 hours, I would be blindsided by nausea, vomiting, cold sweats, fever, bloating, and severe abdominal cramping. Gwen and I wondered if I was the victim of food poisoning.

At 3 a.m. I found myself at the ER with Gwen by my side. The first thing the doctors checked for was, of course, food poisoning. Negative. Next, they looked for a possible intestinal obstruction. These gastrointestinal blockages are not uncommon for Whipple surgery patients. The delicate replumbing of my intestinal tract in April 2007 created odd turns, curves, and angles that complicate digestion and flow. The scar tissue that developed after the reattachment of my stomach, colon, and pancreas simply made matters worse. But, even though this also seemed like a possible cause of my pain and suffering, it wasn't.

I finally got my answer after a CT scan and a blood test that measures lipase enzymes pinpointed an inflamed pancreas. Pancreatitis is yet another complication from my Whipple surgery. The remedy? Lots of bed rest and liquids to give the pancreas a chance to recover. This was accomplished by several days spent in a hospital bed on a strict IV diet with a few sips of water now and again. While I would recover, this incident, combined with my elevated tumor markers, triggered a re-evaluation of my treatment. Instead of keeping an eye on my tumor markers, it was decided that another round of chemotherapy would be the smartest approach.

Of course, this latest setback wasn't the first. In April of 2009, after two years of successfully fighting my disease, I heard the words every cancer patient dreads: Your cancer has returned. Not only had it returned, but it had spread to my lung.

Battling Cancer's Return

During my initial diagnosis, the doctors had discovered that my cancer had metastasized to my colon, abdomen, chest, and neck. This was a huge blow. But two rounds of chemotherapy seemed to rein in its spread. Combined with an aggressive treatment plan that included supplements, diet, and exercise, as well as ongoing acupuncture treatments, the cancer had seemed to be in check. But, now, it looked like the cancer was once again on the move.

Although I was devastated at the return of my cancer almost two years to the date of my initial diagnosis, I refused to give in or give up. I opted for surgery, followed by yet another round of chemo. The procedure, known as a lingulectomy, would remove the quarter-size tumor from my lung. While it might sound complicated, the operation would be child's play compared to the extensive Whipple surgery.

Ultimately, the surgeon ended up removing about 20 percent of my lung along with a nearby lymph node that also harbored cancer. As I was wheeled into the recovery room, my tumor was on its way to the lab for high-tech testing to determine its cancerous nature. It would be tested against a variety of chemo drugs to see which ones would be most effective. This type of futuristic testing is controversial because the tumor is exposed to chemotherapy agents in a test tube rather than the human body. Yet, it was the best way to find out which drugs my tumor might be sensitive to.

Initially, I was told that I could probably go home a couple of days after my surgery. Unfortunately, my lung had other plans. It had developed a small but troublesome air leak. This meant another procedure to remedy the situation. This packed on additional days in the hospital. Finally, however, I was allowed to go home and anxiously await the results of the tumor testing. When the news finally came, our hearts fell again. The tumor was resistant to all of the chemotherapy agents they tried.

Even with this news, chemotherapy was my only option. The tumor had been too close to my heart to safely use radiation, but Dr. Chue and Dr. Cunningham thought that a metronomically dosed combination of the chemotherapy drugs cisplatin and CPT-11 might work. Even though the tumor tested as resistant to cisplatin, it hadn't been tested against CPT-11. I crossed my fingers and began a third round of chemo on June 1, 2009.

Initially, the tumor markers increased, but then began to fall. At the end of 12 weeks, my tumor markers had dropped to a high-normal range—a good sign. Yet this time, I would have just seven months of remission before my tumor markers began creeping up again.

Using the Lessons Learned

All cancer patients fear the worsening or the return of their cancer. It's a silent, yet constant, threat as you try to regain some normalcy in your life. Yet nothing can prepare you for it when it does occur. Emotionally, a recurrence like this can trigger an overwhelming sense of despair. For me, facing yet another round of chemotherapy so soon after the last round is devastating. But I will utilize the strategies I have learned over the past four years to shrug this setback off and gear up for another battle. I will not allow the recurrence to dampen my spirit. I will not go down without a fight—even if it is a fight to the death.

Cancer, by its very nature, is unpredictable and ever-changing. It can send you from high peaks of hope to deep valleys of desolation. Hearing that your cancer is back or that it has spread can trigger shockwaves of fear and hopelessness, not unlike the emotions you felt when

---

A SPOUSE'S PERSPECTIVE: The Quest for Control

Control—everyone wants it, or at least a piece of it. Our professionally trained and experienced medical team has been determined to gain control over Mark's cancer for years now. For the times of remission, their treatments have been successful. For the times of recurrence, their treatments attempt to regulate symptoms and side effects.

This cancer demands full control. Our enemy only plays by one set of rules: its own. It taunts treatments. It has neither regard for human life nor an ounce of respect for Mark's courageous efforts.

Mark practices what he preaches. "Don't worry about things you can't control," he says. He is the hardest worker I know when presented with controllable tasks. Not only are these goals mastered or achieved, but always beyond expectations. Yet Mark's acceptance of things beyond his control paves the way for peace of mind. I, however, remain a work in progress.

I have never liked surprises. I am, by nature, a planner. I like to nail down every detail and know the outcome before I ever embark on any project. Predictability is key. In the recesses of my brain, I keep hoping that some unnamed, unknown authority over cancer, lab results, and treatment outcomes would restore a portion of our lives' predictability, stability, and routine. And yet I find myself living a life of scary suspense.

Whenever I find myself wrestling for control in this out-of-control situation ruled by cancer, I hear the calmness in Mark's reassuring voice: "Gwen, everything will be just fine."

— Gwen

you were first diagnosed. Some people say that a second or third cancer diagnosis can be even more distressing than the first. But, because you have been through this before, you are better equipped to deal with all that a cancer recurrence can bring.

That's not to say that dealing with these feelings is a cakewalk. It's not. In fact, coping with an uptick in your disease may seem like an impossible task. You may find yourself second-guessing the choices you made the first time around. You may wonder if your body is up to the challenge of yet another battle against the disease. You may also be surprised at how intense your emotions are as you contemplate your situation. Don't assume that, just because you've dealt with all of this before, it gets any easier.

Most people, when faced with a recurrence or an unexpected worsening of their cancer experience the following:

* **DISTRESS.** When treatment for the initial cancer ends, it's easy to develop a false sense of security. Most people, including myself, tend to think in a forward motion. You have a problem; you get treated; you get better. End of story. But that's not what often happens with cancer. Nevertheless, the shock of having cancer once again rearing its ugly head can cause distress—sometimes more so than your first diagnosis did.

* **SELF DOUBT.** It's not uncommon to question the treatment plan you chose for your initial diagnosis or the lifestyle choices you've made since your last cancer experience. Do not look backward. Instead, focus on your current situation and what you need to do now to move forward.

* **ANGER.** When cancer returns, you may be angry at the unfairness of it all. You may be angry at the cancer. You may even be angry with your doctor for not eradicating your cancer the first time. As we discussed in Chapter 10, you can use this anger in a positive way to help you fight the resurgence of your cancer.

* **FATIGUE.** It's normal to feel like you simply can't deal with cancer again. Whether it's the side effects of treatment you're dreading or having to tell your friends and family that you have cancer, you've done this all before. You can do it again.

The good news is that the same coping mechanisms you used when you were initially diagnosed with cancer are likely to work again. You also have other advantages to help you deal with the emotional aftershocks this time around. Rely on these to help you cope. For example:

*   **YOU ARE MORE EDUCATED.** Knowing more about your cancer and your treatment options can help reduce your anxiety. Think about how much you knew about cancer at your first diagnosis. This time, you know what your treatment will involve and what side effects might be likely. While they might not be pleasant, at least you don't have the anxiety of the unknown.

*   **YOU'VE BUILT RELATIONSHIPS.** You've worked closely with your doctor, and you know your way around the hospital or clinic. This can make you feel more comfortable. You've also probably built some type of support network, whether it's family, friends, or community support groups. Tapping into this support can help you get through this fight once again.

*   **YOU'VE DONE THIS BEFORE.** Based on your first experience with cancer, you know what's best for you during this time. Whether you needed some time alone or preferred having someone nearby, you can draw on your experience to plan ahead.

Use these experiences to your advantage. They can help you feel more in control when making decisions about your treatment. And don't be afraid to express your feelings to your doctor. The conversation that results can give you a better understanding of your situation, and it can help you make treatment decisions.

When Treatment Doesn't Work

Fortunately, my resolve to fight the cancer is as strong as my will to live and my desire to be here for my family. Of course, I'm also a realist. I know that, at some point, the cancer will likely win. When my cancer no longer responds to treatment, different decisions will need to be made.

When the cancer becomes resistant to treatment, when you have tried everything and it's just not working anymore, it's time to re-evaluate your situation. I am told that this is likely to be the toughest time in the battle with cancer. Some patients want to continue the fight, even if the

When Cancer Comes Back

Your cancer can recur in the same place it was originally located or it can migrate to other parts of your body. Where your cancer recurs depends on your original cancer type and stage. Some cancer types commonly recur in specific areas. Recurrence is divided into three categories.

❋ **Local recurrence.** This means the cancer reappears in the same place it was first found, or very close by. The cancer hasn't spread to the lymph nodes or other parts of the body.

❋ **Regional recurrence.** A regional recurrence occurs in the lymph nodes and tissue located in the vicinity of your original cancer.

❋ **Distant recurrence.** This refers to cancer that has metastasized to areas farther away from where your cancer was first located.

Source: Mayo Clinic (www.mayoclinic.com)

odds are extremely slim that treatment will help. They are willing to deal with the side effects of yet another round of chemo or radiation, even though it is unlikely to help them live any longer.

From a medical perspective, these treatment protocols can be used to help ease other symptoms, even if they will not extend survival. For instance, radiation might be used to help ease bone pain. Chemotherapy might be given to help shrink a tumor that would otherwise obstruct the bowel. But this is not the same as getting treatment to try to cure the cancer. If fighting the cancer is the goal, at some point, you need to ask yourself, "Is it worth it?" Fortunately, I'm not there yet. With any luck, this round of chemotherapy will buy me a good chunk of quality time with my wife and sons.

I know that there will come a time when palliative treatment is quite possibly the best option—not to extend my survival but to improve the quality of my life as much as possible. At some point, I may benefit from hospice care. Many times, this can be given at home. Do I want to put Gwen through that? I'm not sure. She has had to deal with so much already. If not at home, then perhaps a hospital, a nursing home, or even a hospice facility? Fortunately, there will be time for these decisions once we determine whether or not this next round of chemo works. For now, there is hope.

CHAPTER TWELVE

Caregiving: Caring for Your Loved One, Caring for Yourself

When you can lovingly be present to yourself,
your presence to others takes on a deeper quality also.
~ Macrina Wiederkehr

CANCER IS NOT A SOLITARY JOURNEY. There are many people who have walked with me along the way, among them healthcare providers, family, and friends. But the most important person is Gwen—my wife, my best friend, my caregiver.

As difficult as it is to live with cancer, I am firmly convinced that it's even harder to care for someone with cancer. As I've watched Gwen transform into a caregiver, I am amazed at her strength and stamina. No matter what I am going though on this strange journey through cancer, she is with me every step of the way. She is the epitome of grace under pressure.

Taking care of a loved one with cancer is never easy. The demands made of all family caregivers, including Gwen, are enormous. To be on-call around the clock, to organize all aspects of patient home care, to manage every appointment, keep track of all medications, and run a household can be exhausting. But, beyond the physical demands of caregiving, the emotional trials of watching a loved one suffer can be overwhelming.

Even though a couple pledges to care for each other "for better or for worse, in sickness and in health" on their wedding day, nothing can prepare you for the rigors of caregiving. It was certainly not on Gwen's radar the day she married me. But, even though I have benefited from extraordinary medical care, I know I would not be here today if not for the tender, loving, and competent care Gwen provides every minute of every day.

When You Are Called to Give Care

The second your loved one is diagnosed with cancer—or any life-threatening illness—both of your lives are forever changed. As a caregiver, your priorities shift, and your daily routine is suddenly altered. You are now responsible for another human being's welfare. But you are not alone. A 2009 survey found that more than 65 million Americans are the primary caregiver for an adult family member or a child with special needs. It may not be a club you've elected to join, but here you are.

Typical Caregiving Tasks

Here are just a few of the important ways a caregiver can provide invaluable help to the cancer patient:

* Transportation
* Housework
* Grocery shopping
* Food preparation
* Managing finances
* Helping with medication

Many caregivers also must help patients with the tasks of daily living, including:

* Getting in and out of bed
* Getting dressed
* Helping the patient bathe or shower
* Getting to and from the toilet
* Feeding
* Dealing with incontinence and diapers

During those first days, you may be eager to jump right in to your caregiving duties. You may, on the other hand, feel overwhelmed and wonder just where to begin. While each caregiver's situation is unique, everyone shares universal experiences that encompass physical, emotional, and spiritual—not to mention economic and legal—concerns.

In the early stages, most caregivers are focused on the physical chores required of them. However, there are a number of other important tasks caregivers perform on behalf of their loved ones. These include:

* **BEING AS KNOWLEDGEABLE AS POSSIBLE.** By learning about the type of cancer your loved one has—its stage, treatment options, and side effects—you will know what to expect and the right questions to ask. The more you know, the more likely you will be able to spot a problem and alert the other members of the treatment team.

* **GETTING TO KNOW THE CANCER TREATMENT TEAM.** The team typically includes the oncologist and possibly an oncology surgeon and radiologist. Other team members can include an oncology naturopath, acupuncturist, certified herbalist, nutritionist, oncology social workers, mental health experts, nurses, pharmacists, home health aides, rehabilitation specialists, clergy, and hospice care workers. As a member of this team, the caregiver needs to develop positive relationships with these specialists. Have all of their contact numbers and don't be afraid to use them. Ask a lot of questions. If you don't understand the answer, ask the question in another way.

* **ACTING AS AN ADVOCATE.** Look out for your loved one's best interests, not only with the medical team, but with insurance companies, government agencies, and financial institutions. In order to be a better advocate, understand and use the terminology that each group or agency uses in discussing the case. Be calm but firm.

* **MAINTAINING ALL MEDICAL RECORDS.** Keep a current file of all medications (including dosing information) and physicians, along with complete notes on the patient's medical history.

* **KEEPING TRACK OF ALL MEDICATIONS AND SUPPLEMENTS.** Know what each one does and what side effects to look for. You may need to give the cancer patient his or her medications and keep all of the prescriptions up to date.

✳ **GOING TO DOCTOR VISITS WITH YOUR LOVED ONE.** Bring the medical folder to each appointment. Ask questions, take notes, and be a good patient advocate. Let the doctor know about any new symptoms or any other concerns.

✳ **MINIMIZING STRESS.** Treatment for cancer can mean a hectic schedule of doctor's appointments, diagnostic tests, chemotherapy or radiation sessions, and adjunct therapy like acupuncture. Try to reduce stress by simplifying other types of activities, slowing the pace when at home, and ensuring there is plenty of quiet time for recuperation.

Simply keeping up with these tasks can be daunting enough. Add in the day-to-day tasks of working, cooking, cleaning, and keeping a household running smoothly—as well as all of the emotions that accompany

---

Warning Signs of Caregiver Burnout

There is a fine line between being an effective caregiver and being a caregiver who needs help himself. Here are 10 signs you may at risk of becoming a secondary victim to your loved one's disease.

✳ **Being too rigid.** You deal in absolutes and don't give yourself any flexibility. This can set you up for burnout.

✳ **Your friends have stopped calling.** You can alienate friends and acquaintances when all of your conversations begin and end with your loved one's illness. If caregiving dominates your life, you may be pushing your friends away without even realizing it.

✳ **You can't remember the last time you laughed.** It is important to look for positives, whether they are found in lighthearted activities or in humor. Every day needs at least a few happy moments in it.

✳ **You want to "do it all."** Taking on the entire burden of caring for a loved one can be overwhelming. Be willing to let go a little and share the responsibility, at least on occasion.

✳ **You are overweight or out of shape.** Being selflessly devoted to someone else at the expense of your own health is a recipe for

caregiving—and it's not uncommon to find that you are having difficulty coping with your new situation.

Caregiver Burnout

When you are called upon—perhaps suddenly—to be the one person who is ultimately responsible for meeting the needs of someone with serious medical problems, life can feel overwhelming. Most caregivers embark on this journey with loving determination. Yet because of the physical, mental, and emotional demands, a caregiver can easily become the "second victim" of a loved one's illness.

Because of the unrelenting demands a caregiver faces, it's not surprising that they can become physically, spiritually, and emotionally drained. Depression is not uncommon. A study conducted at Yale

---

disaster. To be an effective caregiver, it's important to safeguard your own health and well-being.

* **You don't set aside any "me" time.** While you may feel guilty about taking time away from your loved one, it's important to take periodic breaks to re-energize. Go to dinner with friends, get a massage, or just take a walk by yourself.

* **All conversations turn to caregiving.** This is a clear sign that caregiving has monopolized your life and your relationships.

* **You have no hobbies.** It's important to have an outlet away from caregiving. While stamp-collecting or bird-watching qualify, so do knitting, joining a book club, or taking adult education courses. The only requirement is that it takes you away from caregiving for a period of time.

* **You can't sleep through the night.** If stress is keeping you up at night, you are losing valuable sleep that can help you cope with the demands of caregiving.

* **You dread waking up in the morning.** Caregiving may make life seem like a bad dream at times. But if you find yourself in a funk on a regular basis, you may be suffering from caregiver depression. Seek help or support.

University found that 30 percent of those caring for a terminally ill loved one suffer from major depressive disorder. And former caregivers may not escape the tentacles of this condition after caregiving ends. A recent study found that 41 percent of former caregivers of a spouse with Alzheimer's disease or another form of dementia experienced mild to severe depression up to three years after their spouse had died. Women seem to be at more risk of caregiver depression than men.

But the health problems a caregiver can experience go beyond psychological. If a caregiver focuses solely on her loved one's well-being at the expense of her own, she can become physically ill as well. Research shows that caregiving triggers hormonal changes in the brain and contributes to low-level inflammation. This, in turn, weakens the immune system. One study compared 18 caregivers with 18 non-caregivers at Emory University School of Medicine in Atlanta. The researchers found that the caregivers had fewer T cells, which are white blood cells that search out and destroy infection-causing viruses and bacteria, as well as cancer cells. The study also showed that the more stress the caregivers experienced, the lower their T cell counts were.

Without adequate support and self-care, caregivers can deteriorate with their loved ones, and sometimes even faster. Still, there is hope. Studies show that effective social support networks offer the vital protection to help caregivers thrive and survive the otherwise harrowing experience of caregiving.

Practical Matters

If the physical and emotional aspects of caring for a loved one weren't daunting enough, many people also find themselves having to deal with

Financial Support for Caregivers

In 2006, the US Congress passed the Lifespan Respite Care Act, which established a program to help states develop affordable and high-quality community respite care for family caregivers. At the beginning of 2010, a number of additional financial support measures were under consideration for caregiving, including a tax credit for those who provide family caregiving and increased funding for national caregiver programs.

the financial and legal aspects of caregiving. Fortunately, I had set many financial and legal safeguards in place long before my diagnosis. Unfortunately, many caregivers have to start from scratch and learn about everything from budgeting to investments to Social Security to power of attorney—all in a matter of weeks or months. It can be an intimidating endeavor. Here are a few steps to help you get started and ease this part of the journey.

* **REVIEW BANK AND FINANCIAL ARRANGEMENTS.** Seek help from an accountant or financial planner if you need help sorting everything out.

* **CHECK ON YOUR LOVED ONE'S MEDICAL COVERAGE.** It's important to know what is covered and what is not. Some home healthcare or medical equipment may not be reimbursable. In addition to private insurance, your loved one may also be eligible for Medicare and/or Medicaid or veterans' benefits. Because of recent healthcare reform, insurance issues and policies will be changing over the next few years. Make sure to keep abreast of these changes as they relate to your family's needs.

* **LOOK INTO SOCIAL SECURITY AND PENSION BENEFITS.** Do this as soon as possible since it may take time for these benefits to take effect.

* **PLAN FOR CARE OPTIONS NOW, AND IN THE FUTURE.** There are times when you may need a break and have no one to stay with your loved one. Fortunately, many communities have adult day care services, supplemental home-based care, and respite care to provide temporary help. There may also come a time when you can no longer care for your loved one at home. Finding the right assisted living or long-term care facility, or even a hospice, is important and requires advanced financial planning.

* **CONSULT WITH AN ATTORNEY.** Caregiving involves a number of legal issues that can seem complicated and confusing. Ask family and friends who have been in a similar situation for a referral or recommendation.

* **MAKE SURE YOU HAVE THE LEGAL DOCUMENTS NECESSARY TO PROTECT THE WISHES OF YOUR LOVED ONE.** These include a healthcare

proxy or medical power of attorney, a living will, and a HIPAA (Health Insurance Portability and Accountability Act) release form.

* **LOOK INTO ESTATE PLANNING.** This will allow the patient to determine how her assets and property should be distributed if and when she dies.

* **IF YOU WORK, LOOK INTO FAMILY AND MEDICAL LEAVE, AS WELL AS OPPORTUNITIES FOR TELECOMMUTING, FLEX-TIME, OR JOB SHARING.** Your Human Resources department can help you learn what

---

A SPOUSE'S PERSPECTIVE: Advice from the Trenches

I do not profess to be an expert on ideal strategies for dealing with primary caregiving, but I can honestly and openly share how my husband's stage 4 cancer, surgeries, multiple recurrences, treatments, leadership, and love have affected me and transformed my role within our family. Perhaps my experiences will offer you some small help in dealing with your own situation.

How much has caring for Mark at home changed my life? Prior to his diagnosis, we lived a charmed life. It was the family life I had always dreamed of. Mark and I had a beautiful, shared partnership in parenting with our primary focus centered on the happiness of our sons. Transitioning from this fairy tale life to one filled with periods of suspense and horror has not been easy for this caregiver-in-training. However, if given the opportunity to relive my life, knowing and experiencing the highest of highs and the lowest of lows, would I do it all over again? In a heartbeat!

Early on, I imagined that my role as caregiver would remain constant throughout time. My tunnel vision was focused on whatever task was at hand. Yet, just as there are documented stages in a cancer diagnosis, I've traveled through distinct stages in caregiving.

In the beginning, I was willing to sacrifice everything and anything to help Mark. Of course, I was clueless about what would be required of me and didn't give a second thought to the toll it would take. I simply did what was expected of me. In time, autopilot took over. My days were spent scheduling appointments, attending appointments with Mark, and giving medical care—including emptying drainage bags, flushing drainage tubes, administering injections, and learning

programs, if any, your employer offers if you suddenly find yourself in the role of caregiver.

While it is important to understand the risks and challenges that face caregivers, no one can really understand what it is like to be suddenly thrust into this role better than someone who has been and still is on the frontlines every day. For that we must turn to Gwen, who has cared for me for more than four years with unfailing loyalty, love, and spirit.

---

to care for Mark's PICC line. I also followed up on insurance; paid bills; filed documents; took a crash course in investing; filled and refilled prescriptions; taught our sons to drive; went to the boys' activities, as well as orthodontic and dermatology appointments; shopped for food; cooked said food; and kept the house clean and maintained the yard. If anything broke down—whether it was the dishwasher or the car—it was up to me to make sure it got fixed. I soon discovered that caregiving was like running a marathon each and every day, whether you wanted to or not, whether you were up to it or not, whether you liked it or not.

Over time, I began to grasp the fact that the effort you invest doesn't guarantee success, so it's wise to appreciate life's fleeting moments. I also discovered that letting down my emotional guard can be healing, and that it's okay not to be strong every hour of every day. I realized that recognizing my limitations and attending to my own needs was also important.

Perhaps the biggest challenge for me has been accepting our circumstances. The feelings of utter helplessness are frustrating. The fact that I am unable to fully restore or maintain Mark's health, regardless of the endless amount of effort invested, has been a thorn in my heart. How much human suffering can he tolerate? How much suffering is mandatory for his survival? Yet, despite my frustrations, if the hills along his journey through cancer become too steep, I am here to shoulder his share of the load for as long as it takes. If the turns in suffering are too sharp, my arms will wrap gently around his pain for as long as needed. I am our family's caregiver and my role is to give care.

SENSE AND SORROW

Once I became an official caregiver, a new sense beyond the basic five senses of sight, hearing, smell, taste, and touch became heightened. A keen awareness of our reality was born.

Seeing sweethearts holding hands is a bittersweet reminder of how my hand once had a home in Mark's. It's a reminder of how the cruel chemo-induced neuropathy has put an end to our hand-holding connection. One of the most basic forms of healing, the human touch, now causes Mark physical pain. For me, it causes heartbreaking pain.

It's the little things I miss, the things most people take for granted, like handholding and cuddling. But we have each other and, for now, that is enough.

I find it disturbing when I see a couple bickering over the most inconsequential things. It is concerning when I run across those who tend to blow what I would consider minor problems out of proportion. I was recently reminded of this when I unintentionally overheard a woman behind me in line at the pharmacy telling her friend about the trials of her hectic life.

"My life is so busy. I'm working on the school's science fair, and I still have to register our family for the Jingle Bell Run. It's just been nonstop. I really do need a few days to relax."

Half annoyed, half amused, I realized that if she knew the flipside of good health, all that negativity would have been quickly silenced. In reality, she had nothing life-threatening to complain about. Although I try to avoid this type of negativity from strangers, it inevitably seeps in to my consciousness on occasion. Fortunately, this is balanced by dozens of small, yet meaningful, acts of kindness every day. Considerate words and deeds are instantly recognized and magnified. Courteous actions boost my faith and stamina. I can still count my blessings. I choose to be thankful.

MANY HATS, ONE BODY

Many spouses become caregivers later in life. Because Mark was so young when he was diagnosed, I found myself adding the demanding role of caregiver to that of wife and mother. Yet, to do so has created unavoidable gaps as a parent. Having to choose Mark's needs over our sons' wishes leaves me with a permanent sense of guilt. James and Lane have been accepting of my absence at school and social activities and sporting events. They understand that my once-full attention and attendance are not always possible these days.

Thankfully, our boys are past the age that requires full-time custodial care. Both James and Lane had learned many of the tools needed to care for themselves—doing laundry, ironing, and basic cooking—prior to their father's diagnosis. That was one less transition to be made. There were other activities that required adult supervision and guidance. For instance, I never imagined that I would be the one who would teach James and Lane to drive. Somehow we all survived and ultimately produced two accomplished licensed drivers.

Juggling all of these roles can, at times, leave me drained. But the support of family and friends has kept me standing. During Mark's series of hospitalizations, Betty, Patti, Fay, and Cousin Ed helped me cover consecutive 24-hour shifts. Thanks to their help, Mark did not have to wait for nursing assistance to maneuver his IV lines or monitor cords, drainage tubes, and bags. Someone was always there to help adjust his deep-vein thrombosis leggings or help him move in and out of bed as his painful surgical incisions healed. Their helping hands allowed me spend afternoons and evenings at home with James and Lane.

In addition to this core team of altruistic family members, my loving parents, Ken and Sarah, have provided weekly meals, transportation, and family care. We are also so grateful to have received the healing thoughts and prayers from siblings, aunts, uncles, cousins, friends, neighbors, and coworkers in multiple ways. And then there is Mark's brilliant team of oncologists, nurses, gastroenterologists, pulmonologists, and surgeons. They have become like family.

While I longed to continue a sense of normalcy and independence, I knew that battling this cancer and keeping our sons' schedules running required much, much more than what I could solely provide. A lengthy list of generous home chefs have prepared and delivered complete dinners when my own thoughts of menus, grocery shopping, and cooking were overwhelmed with Mark's surgeries, treatments, and appointments. Their extended hands have enabled James and Lane to maintain a significant portion of their social lives. They have helped our sons maintain balance and a fair share of fond childhood memories. Family and friends not in the Seattle area have sent compassionate words and heartwarming care packages. Their support carries our hearts from miles away. The outpouring of love we've received in the form of phone calls, cards, emails, visits, meals, transportation, and last-minute favors must be credited for our family's cancer survival. These giving souls are my peacemakers. I have counted on them when my own capable limits have been maximized. When time and energy allow, we plan to continue the cycle of unconditional support by paying it all forward.

THE TOLL OF CAREGIVING

I am sometimes asked how I deal with the negative emotions—the anger, depression, frustration, grief, and guilt—that are inevitable as a long-term caregiver. It helped immensely when I learned that these reactions and feelings were perfectly normal. It also helped to develop a circle of fellow spousal caregivers who openly share their own range of experiences and emotions with me. I know that I am not alone.

Oddly, I have discovered that these emotional stages have had to run their course for me to finally find peace. But it's not a permanent condition. At my annual physical exam, I was told that long-term caregiver stress is not unlike post-traumatic stress syndrome. I am not surprised. Looking back at how much ground our family has covered during our journey with cancer is disturbing. Looking ahead and making plans for the future can be a setup for disappointment.

As difficult as the emotional side of caregiving can be, I must still do the things that need to be done to make sure Mark and the boys are cared for. To keep up with these nonstop demands, I must make sure that I also nurture my own needs, rely on our family's support system, turn to outside resources and, above all, count my blessings. One resource that helps me maintain a healthy perspective is Cancer Lifeline, a Seattle-based hotline that provides emotional support, resources, educational classes, and exercise programs to cancer patients and survivors, as well as caregivers and family members. It's a place where I can anonymously drop the mask of strength and courage and let my emotions flow freely.

I also have a book on my nightstand, as well as an audio CD, that provide consolation. *Daily Comforts for Caregivers* by Pat Samples is a wonderful book that devotes each page to a common challenge and ends with an affirmation. Because each topic takes up only one page, I find that it fits into my busy schedule. *Affirmations* by Belleruth Naperstek is an audio CD that allows me to accept my limitations in caregiving. As I slowly recite these affirmations aloud as directed, they permit me to think of myself and remind me to be my own caregiver.

TAKE A BREAK

If you are a caregiver, do not underestimate the importance of taking time for yourself. These breaks can rejuvenate your stamina and help you be a better caregiver. Although caregivers do not always have the luxury of deciding the timing or duration of any given break, you can decide for yourself what provides the most stress-relief benefits. Along with figuring out what forms of downtime work best for you, don't be shy in asking your support network for help. Relying on your primary support system can afford you the precious time away from your responsibilities.

I have learned firsthand that overextending myself can cause a temporary decline in my own physical health. Once my needs are addressed, however, I can provide the caregiving required to meet the needs of my family. While every caregiver finds relief from different sources, here is what works for me.

* A nap

* Getting in a cardio workout

* Saying a prayer

* Calling my sister, Fay

* Connecting with other caregivers

* Writing in my journal

* Listening to James and Lane play the piano.

The physical, mental, and emotional toll caregiving takes really hit home during my first year of caring for Mark. I unintentionally lost weight and found myself exhausted. Now, in my fourth year of caregiving, I try not to overextend myself during the day. I try to reserve my strength in case my caregiving is needed in the middle of the night. Pacing myself is key. So is getting an adequate amount of sleep. While I can't always get a full night's sleep, particularly before and after Mark's surgeries and while he is undergoing chemotherapy, I nap whenever I can.

Any form of exercise provides tremendous stress relief. It's the bonding agent for my mental, emotional, and spiritual well-being. I look forward to my daily aerobic or yoga DVD workouts and logging time on the treadmill. Not only does exercise strengthen my physical stamina, it helps me feel empowered.

Remembering to eat—and eat sensibly—is also important. I have come to view food as energy and make it a point to eat at least three healthy meals a day. I also try to stay hydrated. I drink six to eight glasses of water daily and avoid caffeine and energy drinks.

While none of this advice is new, it's information that can easily be forgotten in the whirlwind of activity that occurs when you become a caregiver. What you might not think of is the mental and emotional toll caregiving takes. I have learned to avoid negativity, whether it's from the media, current events, or blogs. Instead, I try to surround myself with positivity and encouragement. Periodically, I see an oncology caregiver counselor at the same clinic that serves Mark. While Mark receives a chemotherapy or acupuncture treatment down the hallway, I meditate, discuss life, and practice relaxation and coping techniques with my mind-body therapist.

Writing is another outlet. It provides opportunities for expression. The power in seeing my private thoughts and emotions in printed form is liberating. I feel as though my voice was heard and I am able to move on.

SILVER LININGS

Caregiving is the most mentally and physically exhausting labor of love that I have ever undertaken. Despite all of the challenges, I can smile knowing that Mark and I have spent more time with each other since his diagnosis than at any other period in our 29 years together. Regardless of the activity, it is considered date time with my best friend. Our trust that God is by our side throughout this journey and knowing that we will see our loved ones beyond this life on Earth delivers incredible serenity.

This may not be a chapter I envisioned for our family's story, but it's still a wonderful, wonderful life filled with faith, happiness, and love. And, even though caregiving is a merciless beat set by an unrelenting cancer, it's essential to always be mindful of the important things in life: family, the realization that time is paramount, and the capacity to cherish every moment.

If life and circumstances call upon you to be a caregiver, remember to nurture yourself and know that you are making a positive difference. The task is not easy, but continue loving the one you are caring for and live a hopeful life.

I wish you peace.

— Gwen

Resources

Books

CANCER AND HEALTH

Alschuler, Lise N. and Karolyn A. Gazella. *Alternative Medicine Magazine's Definitive Guide to Cancer: An Integrated Approach to Prevention, Treatment, and Healing.* Berkeley, Calif.: Celestial Arts, 2010 (third edition paperback).

Anderson, Gary. *Cancer: 50 Essential Things to Do.* New York: Plume, 2009.

Block, Keith and Andrew Weil. *Life Over Cancer: The Block Center Program for Integrative Cancer Treatment.* New York: Bantam Dell, 2009.

Bollinger, Ty. *Cancer: Step Outside the Box.* West Conshohocken, Pa.: Infinity, 2006.

Gomez, Isidro. *5,001 Reasons To Survive Pancreatic Cancer: A Motivation Book.* Washington D.C.: Black Mesa Publishing, 2009.

Murray, Michael, Birdsall Tim, Pizzorno JE, and Reilly Paul. *How To Prevent and Treat Cancer with Natural Medicine.* New York: Riverhead Books. 2002.

O'Reilly, Eileen and Joanne Frankel Kelvin. *100 Questions & Answers About Pancreatic Cancer.* Sudbury, Mass.: Jones and Bartlett, 2009.

Pausch, Randy and Jeffrey Zaslow. *The Last Lecture.* New York: Hyperion, 2008.

Pescatore, Fred and Karolyn Gazella. *Boost Your Health with Bacteria.* El Segundo, California: Active Interest Media, 2009.

U.S. Government. *Pancreatic Cancer Toolkit – Comprehensive Medical Encyclopedia with Treatment Options, Clinical Data, and Practical Information* (CD). Progressive Management, 2009.

CAREGIVING

American Medical Association. *American Medical Association Guide to Home Caregiving.* New York: Wiley, 2001.

Canfield, Jack, Mark Victor Hansen, LeAnn Thieman. *Chicken Soup for the Caregiver's Soul: Stories to Inspire Caregivers in the Home, the Community and the World.* Deerfield Beach, Fla.: HCI Books, 2004.

Hennessey Maya. *If Only I'd Had This Caregiving Book.* Bloomington, Indiana: AuthorHouse, 2006.

Meyer, Maria and Paula Derr. *The Comfort of Home: A Complete Guide for Caregivers.* Portland, Ore.: CareTrust Publications, 2007.

Naperstek, Belleruth. *Affirmations.* New York: Image Paths, 1995. [Audio CD]

Samples, Pat. *Daily Comforts for Caregivers.* Minneapolis: Fairview Press, 1999.

Sheehy, Gail. *Passages In Caregiving.* New York: William Morrow, 2010.

Strom, Kay Marshall. *A Caregiver's Survival Guide: How to Stay Healthy When Your Loved One Is Sick.* Westmont, Ill.: InterVarsity Press, 2000.

HEALTHY COOKBOOKS

Jenkins, Nancy Harmon. *The New Mediterranean Diet Cookbook.* New York: Bantam Dell, 2009.

Katz, R and Mat Edelson. *The Cancer-Fighting Kitchen: Nourishing, Big-Flavor Recipes for Cancer Treatment and Recovery.* Berkeley, Calif.: Celestial Arts, 2009.

La Puma, Steve and Rebecca Powell Marx. *Chef MD's Big Book of Culinary Medicine.* New York: Crown Publishers. 2008.

Larson, A and Ivy Larson. *Whole Foods Diet Cookbook.* Layton, Utah: Gibbs Smith, 2009.

Mathai, K and Ginny Smith. *The Cancer Lifeline Cookbook: Recipes, Ideas, and Advice to Optimize the Lives of People Living with Cancer.* Seattle: Sasquatch Books, 2004.

Miletello, Gerald and Holly Clegg. *Eating Well Through Cancer: Easy Recipes & Recommendations During & After Treatment.* Memphis, Tenn.: Wimmer, 2001.

Petusevsky, Steve. *The Whole Foods Market Cookbook.* New York: Clarkson Potter, 2002.

Reno, Tosca. *Tosca Reno's Eat Clean Cookbook.* Ontario, Canada: Robert Kennedy Publishing, 2009.

The Moosewood Collective. *Moosewood Restaurant Low-Fat Favorites.* New York: Clarkson Potter, 1996.

Weihofen, Donna. *The Cancer Survival Cookbook: 200 Quick & Easy Recipes with Helpful Eating Hints.* New York: Wiley, 1997.

Weil, Andrew and Rosie Daley. *The Healthy Kitchen.* New York: Alfred A. Knopf. 2002.

MINDFULNESS

Dalai Lama. *The Art of Happiness.* New York: Riverhead Hardcover. 2009.

Kabat-Zinn, Jon. *Full Catastrophe Living: Using the Wisdom of Your Body and Mind to Face Stress, Pain, and Illness.* Brooklyn, NY: Delta Publishing Group. 1990.

Nhat Hanh, Thich. *Peace Is Every Step: The Path of Mindfulness in Everyday Life.* New York: Bantam. 1992.

Caregiver Resources

Family Caregiver Alliance
180 Montgomery St., Suite 1100
San Francisco, CA 94104
Phone: 800-445-8106

Web site: www.caregiver.org

The Family Caregiver Alliance (FCA), provides information and support to caregivers, publishes fact sheets about caregiving issues in English, Spanish, and Chinese. The organization also offers advice about how to handle caregiving responsibilities and the health impacts that stress can have on caregivers. It also provides online support groups.

National Family Caregivers Association
10400 Connecticut Avenue, Suite 500
Kensington, MD 20895-3944
Phone: 800-896-3650

Web site: www.thefamilycaregiver.org

The National Family Caregivers Association educates, supports, empowers, and speaks up for the more than 50 million Americans who care for loved ones with a chronic illness or disability or the frailties of old age. This organization also provides information and resources for caregivers and connects caregivers with each other to provide emotional and spiritual support.

Well Spouse Association
63 West Main Street, Suite H
Freehold, NJ 07728
Phone: 800-838-0879

Web site: www.wellspouse.org

A nonprofit organization founded in 1988 by author and spousal caregiver, Maggie Strong, whose husband was diagnosed with multiple sclerosis (MS). Today, the Well Spouse provides emotional peer-to-peer support to the wives, husbands, and partners of the chronically ill and/or disabled.

Cancer Education Web sites

American Cancer Society
Web site: www.cancer.org

A nationwide, community-based, voluntary health organization that provides information on all types of cancer. It also sponsors research and community programs in cancer prevention and management.

ChemoCare
Web site: www.chemocare.com

Created as an educational partnership between former Olympic ice skater and cancer survivor Scott Hamilton and the Cleveland Clinic Cancer Center, this site offers a wealth of information on traditional chemotherapy, including information on a wide variety of chemotherapy drugs. It also provides tips for managing the effects of chemo as well as inspirational stories from survivors.

The National Cancer Institute

Web site: www.cancer.gov

Part of the National Institutes of Health of the United States Department of Health and Human Services, the National Cancer Institute is the federal Government's principal agency for cancer research. The National Cancer Institute conducts, coordinates, and funds cancer research, training, health information dissemination, and other programs on the cause, diagnosis, prevention, and treatment of cancer.

National Center for Complementary and Alternative Medicine

Web site: http://nccam.nih.gov

A federal agency that uses science to explore complementary and alternative medicine (CAM) practices, trains CAM researchers, and provides authoritative information about CAM to professionals and the public. NCCAM awards grants for research projects, training, and career development in CAM; sponsors conferences, educational programs, and exhibits; studies ways to use proven CAM practices along with conventional medical practice; and supports adding CAM to medical, dental, and nursing school programs. NCCAM is part of the National Institutes of Health.

National Institutes of Health

Web site: www.nih.gov

A federal agency in the United States that conducts biomedical research in its own laboratories; supports the research of non-federal scientists in universities, medical schools, hospitals, and research institutions throughout the country and abroad; helps in the training of research investigators; and fosters communication of medical information.

The National Pancreas Foundation

101 Federal Street, Suite 1900
Boston, MA 02110
Phone: 866-726-2737

Web site: www.pancreasfoundation.org

Provides information and support to patients with pancreatic cancer. This organization also raises money for research into better screening and treatment for the disease and ultimately a cure.

The Oncology Channel

Web site: www.oncologychannel.com

Developed and monitored by board-certified physicians, The Oncology Channel provides comprehensive information about tumors, the various types of cancer, and cancer treatments.

WebMD

Web site: www.webmd.com

An easy-to-understand yet in-depth source of information on all types of diseases, including cancer. Content includes health news, an up-to-date medical reference database, medical imagery and animation, live web events, interactive tools, and more.

Integrative Medicine Referrals and Resources

American Association of Integrative Physicians
2750 East Sunshine
Springfield, MO 65804
Phone: 877-718-3053
Web site: www.aaimedicine.com

Promotes the development of integrative medicine. The Web site provides a searchable database of integrative healthcare providers.

American Association of Naturopathic Physicians
4435 Wisconsin Avenue, NW, Suite 403
Washington, DC 20016
Phone: 202-237-8150
Web site: www.naturopathic.org

A national professional society representing licensed or licensable naturopathic physicians. It provides patients with information on naturopathy and offers a searchable database of qualified naturopaths.

American College for Advancement in Medicine
8001 Irvine Center Drive, Suite 825
Irvine, CA 92618
Phone: 800-532-3688
Web site: www.acamnet.org

Provides information on integrative medicine, as well as various medical conditions and treatments. The Web site also offers a searchable database of integrative physicians.

Cancer Treatment Centers of America
1336 Basswood Road
Schaumburg, IL 60173
Phone: 800-268-0786
Web site: www.cancercenter.com

Oncology Association of Naturopathic Physicians
216 NE Fremont St.
Portland, OR 97212
Phone: 800-490-8509

A professional association of naturopathic physicians who work with cancer patients in a holistic way using natural medicines, foods and lifestyle changes.

Dietary Supplements

Supplements obtained through your healthcare provider

Biotics Research Corp.
6801 Biotics Research Drive
Rosenberg, TX 77471
Phone: 800-231-5777
Web site: www.bioticsresearch.com

Specially designed, high-potency nutritional supplements, including vitamin D and fish oil.

Thorne Research
25820 Highway 2 West
Sandpoint, ID 83864
Phone: 800-228-1966

Web site: www.thorne.com

Condition-focused hypoallergenic supplements made without additives, flowing agents, or binders.

Over-the-counter supplements

Dr. Ohhira's Essential Formulas, Inc.
P.O. Box 166139
Irving, TX 75016
Phone: 972-255-3918

Web site: www.essentialformulas.com

Probiotics developed during a natural temperature fermentation process that contain 12 strains of live lactic acid bacteria, 4 organic acids, 10 vitamins, 8 minerals, 18 amino acids, naturally occurring fructooligosaccharide (FOS).

EuroMedica USA
955 Challenger Drive
Green Bay WI 54311
Phone: 866-598-5487

Web site: www.euromedicausa.com

A wide range of supplements that benefit cancer patients, including curcumin, immune-stimulating blends, and a whole-foods omega-3 complex.

New Chapter
90 Technology Drive
Brattleboro, VT 05301
Phone: 800-543-7279

Web site: www.newchapter.com

A variety of whole-foods supplements that target inflammation and immunity using supercritical extracts. These include medicinal mushrooms, whole-foods fish oil, and full-spectrum turmeric.

Wakunaga of America/Kyolic Aged Garlic Extract
23501 Madero
Mission Viejo, CA 92691
Phone: 800-421-2998

Web site: www.kyolic.com

More than 620 scientific studies support the health benefits of Kyolic Aged Garlic Extract (AGE). Odorless and non-irritating, research shows that AGE protects the immune system—specifically natural killer cell activity—during times of stress. Kyolic also creates aged garlic blends geared toward specific conditions as well as whole-foods green supplements, chlorella, and probiotic blends.

Mind-Body Resources

American Association of Acupuncture and Oriental Medicine
PO Box 162340
Sacramento, CA 95816
Phone: 866-455-7999
Web site: www.aaaomonline.org

Provides patient information as well as a searchable database of qualified, licensed acupuncturists.

Association for Applied Psychophysiology and Biofeedback
10200 W. 44th Avenue, Suite 304
Wheat Ridge, CO 80033-2840
Phone: 800-422-8436
Web site: www.aapb.org

Along with a wealth of information on biofeedback and the conditions it can help to treat, the Web site provides helpful information on insurance issues as well as the best way to locate a provider.

American Massage Therapy Association
500 Davis Street, Suite 900
Evanston, IL 60201-4695
Phone: 877-905-2700
Web site: www.amtamassage.org

Offers a consumer guide to massage and a searchable database of trained and certified massage therapists.

Patient Advocacy

CancerCare
275 Seventh Avenue
New York, NY 10001
Phone: 800-813-4673
Web site: www.cancercare.org

Provides counseling, online and telephone support, educational information, and financial assistance to patients, families, and caregivers who are dealing with all types of cancer. The organization offers specialized programs that focus on the unique needs of caregivers, children and young adults, patients with rare or advanced cancers, and individuals facing end-of-life issues. CancerCare's services are available in English and Spanish. Programs are provided by trained oncology social workers and are completely free of charge.

Cancer Hope Network
2 North Road, Suite A
Chester, NJ 07930
Phone: 877-467-3638
Web site: www.cancerhopenetwork.org

Provides free and confidential one-on-one support to cancer patients and their families. All support volunteers are specially trained cancer survivors.

Lance Armstrong Foundation
P.O. Box 161150
Austin, TX 78716
Phone: 866-467-7205
Web site: www.livestrong.org

Seeks to promote the optimal physical, psychological, and social recovery and care of cancer survivors and their loved ones. The LAF focuses its activities on survivorship education and resources, community programs, national advocacy initiatives, and scientific and clinical research grants. The organization's Web site features a variety of information and resources for people living with cancer.

Marti Nelson Cancer Foundation
1520 East Covell Blvd., Suite B5103
Davis, CA 95616
Phone: 530-756-0291
Web site: www.canceractionnow.org

Works to make effective and safe cancer treatments available to cancer patients. The Web site provides information on standard and non-standard treatment options, clinical trials, and experimental drugs. The organization is volunteer-driven and provides its services free of charge.

Patient Advocate Foundation
700 Thimble Shoals Blvd, Suite 200
Newport News, VA 23606
Phone: 800-532-5274
Web site: www.patientadvocate.org

Provides mediation and arbitration services on behalf of patients with chronic, debilitating, and life-threatening illnesses regarding problems with their medical bills, insurance, and employment.

The Center for Patient Partnerships
975 Bascom Mall, Suite 4311
Madison, WI 53706
Phone: 608-265-6267
Web site: http://patientpartnerships.org

An advocacy and education program that advocates for the needs and rights of people facing life-threatening diseases, including cancer, all around the world. The Center for Patient Partnerships helps patients understand their diagnoses and treatment options, deal with illness-related work issues, and handle insurance issues.

Research

PubMed
US National Library of Medicine
8600 Rockville Pike
Bethesda, MD 20894
Web site: www.ncbi.nlm.nih.gov/pubmed

A searchable database of more than 19 million peer-reviewed published studies from MEDLINE and life science journals.

Support Groups

Cancer Lifeline
6522 Fremont Ave. North
Seattle, WA 98103
Phone: 800-255-5505

Web site: www.cancerlifeline.org

This Seattle-based program provides emotional support, resources, education, and exercise programs that are designed to support cancer patients, their friends and family, and caregivers. These services are available throughout the Puget Sound area and in 16 western Washington counties.

Pancreatic Cancer Action Network
2141 Rosecrans Ave., Suite 7000
El Segundo, CA 90245
Phone: 877-272-6226

Web site: www.pancan.org

A national organization creating hope in a comprehensive way through research, patient support, community outreach, and advocacy for a cure.

Pancreatic Cancer Alliance
Web site: www.pancreaticalliance.org

A clearinghouse of support groups online and around America.

Glossary

A diagnosis of cancer can make it seem like you've been transported to another country. Too often, doctors and other healthcare providers sound like they are speaking a foreign language. Here is a "cheat sheet" to help you decipher some of the medical terms you may hear.

Ablation: This refers to the removal or destruction of an organ or tissue. Ablation may be performed by surgery, hormones, drugs, radiofrequency, heat, or other methods.

Abnormal: Not normal. An abnormal lesion or growth may be cancerous, premalignant (likely to become cancer), or benign (not cancer).

Active Surveillance: Closely monitoring a patient's condition but withholding treatment until symptoms appear or change. This is also called observation or watchful waiting.

Acupressure: The application of pressure or manipulation to specific acupoints on the body to control symptoms such as pain or nausea. It is a type of complementary and alternative medicine.

Acupuncture: Inserting thin needles into the skin at specific points (acupoints) on the body to control pain, nausea, and other symptoms. Can be used as an adjunct to chemotherapy or radiation.

Acute: Symptoms or signs that begin and worsen quickly; not chronic.

Adenocarcinoma: Cancer that begins in cells that line certain internal organs and that have gland-like (secretory) properties.

Amylase: An enzyme that helps the body digest starches.

Ampulla: A sac-like enlargement of a canal or duct.

Ampulla of Vater: The place where the common bile duct is connected to the small intestine.

Ampullary Cancer: Cancer that forms in the ampulla of Vater (an enlargement of the ducts from the liver and pancreas where they join and enter the small intestine). Symptoms include jaundice, abdominal pain, nausea, vomiting, and weight loss. Also called ampulla of Vater cancer.

Antagonist: In medicine, a substance that stops the action or effect of another substance. For example, a drug that blocks the stimulating effect of estrogen on a tumor cell is called an estrogen receptor antagonist.

Antibody: A protein made by plasma cells (a type of white blood cell) in response to an a substance that causes the body to make a specific immune response (antigen). Each antibody can bind to only one specific antigen and its goal is to annihilate that antigen. Some antibodies destroy antigens directly. Others make it easier for white blood cells to destroy the antigen.

Antigen: Any substance that causes the body to make a specific immune response.

Apoptosis: A type of cell death in which a series of molecular steps in a cell leads to its death. This is the body's normal way of getting rid of unneeded or abnormal cells. The process of apoptosis may be blocked in cancer cells. Also called programmed cell death.

Benign: Not cancerous. Benign tumors may grow larger but do not spread to other parts of the body. Also called nonmalignant.

Bile: A digestive juice secreted by the liver and stored in the gallbladder that aids in the digestion of fats.

Bile Duct: A tube that carries bile from the liver to the gallbladder and then to the small intestine.

Bile Salts: Conjugates (protein that contains both amino and non-amino acids) of glycine or taurine with bile acids. These are formed in the liver and secreted in the bile. They are powerful detergents that break down fat globules, enabling them to be digested.

Biliary Tree: The path by which bile is secreted by the liver on its way to the duodenum or small intestine. It is called a tree because it begins with many small branches which end in the common bile duct.

Bilirubin: A yellowish-orange substance that is made by the normal break-down of red blood cells. It is broken down by the liver and leaves the body in the stools. Extra bilirubin in the blood causes jaundice, which is a yellowing of the skin.

Biomarker: A molecule found in blood, other body fluids, or tissues that is a sign of a normal or abnormal process, or of a condition or disease. A biomarker may be used to see how well the body responds to a treatment for a disease or condition.

Biopsy: The removal of cells or tissues for examination by a pathologist. The pathologist may study the tissue under a microscope or perform other tests on the cells or tissue. There are many different types of biopsy procedures. The most common include: (1) incisional biopsy, in which only a sample of tissue is removed; (2) excisional biopsy, in which an entire lump or suspicious area is removed; and (3) needle biopsy, in which a sample of tissue or fluid is removed with a needle. When a wide needle is used, the procedure is called a core biopsy. When a thin needle is used, the procedure is called a fine-needle aspiration biopsy.

C-Peptide: A substance made by the pancreas. C-peptide and insulin are both part of a larger molecule that gets split apart before being released into the blood. Abnormal blood levels of C-peptide may occur in certain diseases, such as diabetes or cancer.

Cancer: A term used for diseases in which abnormal cells divide uncontrollably and can spread to nearby tissues. Cancer cells can also make their way to other parts of the body through the blood and lymph systems. There are more than 200 different types of cancer and most fall within five categories. Carcinoma is a cancer that begins in the skin or in tissues that line internal organs. Sarcoma is a cancer that begins in bone, cartilage, fat, muscle, blood vessels or other connective or supportive tissue. Leukemia is a cancer that starts in blood-forming tissue such as the bone marrow. Lymphoma and multiple myeloma are cancers that begin in the cells of the immune system. Central nervous system cancers are cancers that begin in the tissues of the brain and spinal cord. Pancreatic cancer is considered a carcinoma.

Capillary: The smallest type of blood vessel. A capillary connects small arteries to small veins. This creates a network of blood vessels throughout the body. The wall of a capillary is thin and leaky, and capillaries are involved in the exchange of fluids and gases between tissues and the blood.

Carcinoma in Situ: A group of abnormal cells that remain in the place where they first formed. They have not spread. These abnormal cells may become cancer and spread into nearby normal tissue. Also called stage 0 disease.

Carcinogen: Any substance that causes cancer.

Carcinoma: Cancer that begins in the skin or in tissues that line or cover internal organs.

Cell: The individual unit that makes up the tissues of the body. All living things are made up of one or more cells.

Cell Cycle: The process a cell goes through each time it divides. The cell cycle consists of a series of steps during which the chromosomes and other cell material double to make two copies. The cell then divides into two daughter cells, each receiving one copy of the doubled material. The cell cycle is complete when each daughter cell is surrounded by its own outer membrane.

Cell Proliferation: An increase in the number of cells as a result of cell growth and cell division.

Cell Respiration: A chemical process in which oxygen is used to make energy from carbohydrates (sugars).

Chemotherapy: Treatment with drugs that kill cancer cells.

Chinese Meridian Theory: In traditional Chinese medicine, meridians are channels that form a network in the body, through which qi (vital energy) flows. Blocked qi causes pain or illness. The flow of qi is restored by using pressure, needles, suction or heat at hundreds of specific points along the meridians.

Chronic: A disease or condition that persists or progresses over a long period of time.

Clinical Trial: A type of research study that tests how well new medical approaches work in people. These studies test new methods of screening, prevention, diagnosis or treatment of a disease.

Complementary and Alternative Medicine (CAM): Specific types of natural treatments that are used in addition to (complementary) or instead of (alternative) standard treatments. CAM may include dietary supplements, herbal preparations, special teas, acupuncture, massage therapy, magnet therapy, spiritual healing, and meditation.

Cytokine: Various protein molecules secreted by cells of the immune system that serve to regulate the immune system.

Dietary Reference Intakes: A set of guidelines developed by U.S. and Canadian scientists to give information about the role of nutrients in human health. These guidelines include the Reference Daily Intakes (RDI), which are the recommended amounts of nutrients to be eaten each day to prevent deficiency. This system replaced the Recommended Dietary Allowances (RDA). Also called DRI.

Dietary Supplement: A nutritional product that is added to the diet. A dietary supplement is taken by mouth, and usually contains one or more ingredients such as vitamins, minerals, herbs, amino acids, and enzymes). Also called nutritional supplement.

Differentiation: In cancer, this refers to how well-developed the cancer cells are in a tumor. Differentiated tumor cells resemble normal cells and tend to grow and spread at a slower rate than undifferentiated or poorly differentiated tumor cells, which lack the structure and function of normal cells and grow uncontrollably.

Distal: In medicine, refers to a part of the body that is farther away from the center of the body than another part. For example, the fingers are distal to the shoulder. The opposite is proximal.

Distal Pancreatectomy: Removal of the body and tail of the pancreas.

Dose Dependent: Refers to the effects of treatment with a drug. If the effects change when the dose of the drug is changed, the effects are said to be dose-dependent.

Doubling Time: In biology, the amount of time it takes for one cell to divide or for a group of cells (such as a tumor) to double in size. The doubling time is different for different kinds of cancer cells or tumors.

Drug Resistance: The failure of cancer cells, viruses or bacteria to respond to a drug used to kill or weaken them. The cells, viruses or bacteria may be resistant to the drug at the beginning of treatment, or may become resistant after being exposed to the drug.

Early-Stage Cancer: A term used to describe cancer that is early in its growth, and may not have spread to other parts of the body. What is called early stage may differ between cancer types.

Efficacy: In medicine, the ability of a treatment technique to produce the desired beneficial effect.

Endocrine: Tissue that makes and releases hormones that travel in the bloodstream and control the actions of other cells or organs. Some examples of endocrine tissues are the pituitary, thyroid, and adrenal glands.

Endocrine Pancreas Cell: A pancreatic cell that produces hormones (e.g., insulin and glucagon) that are secreted into the bloodstream. These hormones help control the level of glucose (sugar) in the blood. Also called islet cell and islet of Langerhans cell.

Endogenous: Produced inside an organism or cell. The opposite is external (exogenous) production.

Enteral Nutrition: Nutrition that is delivered into the digestive system as a liquid. Drinking nutrition beverages or formulas and tubefeeding are forms of enteral nutrition. People who are unable to meet their needs with food and beverages alone, and who experience vomiting or uncontrollable diarrhea may be given tubefeedings. Tubefeeding can be used to add to what a person is able to eat or can be the only source of nutrition. A small feeding tube may be placed through the nose into the stomach or the small intestine, or it may be surgically placed into the stomach or the intestinal tract through an opening made on the outside of the abdomen, depending on how long it will be used.

Enzyme: A protein that speeds up chemical reactions in the body.

Exocrine Cancer: A disease in which malignant (cancer) cells are found in the tissues of the pancreas. Also called pancreatic cancer.

Exocrine Pancreas Cell: A pancreatic cell that produces enzymes that are secreted into the small intestine. These enzymes help digest food as it passes through the gastrointestinal tract.

External-Beam Radiation Therapy: A type of radiation therapy that uses a machine to aim high-energy rays at the cancer from outside of the body. Also called external radiation therapy.

False Positive: A test result that indicates that a person has a specific disease or condition when the person actually does not have the disease or condition.

Fibroblast: A connective tissue cell that makes and secretes collagen proteins.

Free Radical: An atom that has at least one unpaired electron. Free radicals are highly reactive and can damage important cellular molecules such as DNA or lipids or other parts of the cell.

Gallbladder: A pear-shaped organ just below the liver that stores the bile secreted by the liver. During a fatty meal, the gallbladder contracts, delivering the bile through the bile ducts into the intestines to help with digestion.

Gastric Feeding Tube: A tube that is inserted through the nose, down the throat and esophagus, and into the stomach. It can be used to give drugs, liquids, and liquid food, or used to remove substances from the stomach. Giving food through a gastric feeding tube is a type of enteral nutrition. Also called nasogastric tube and NG tube.

Gastrointestinal Tract: The stomach and intestines. The gastrointestinal tract is part of the digestive system, which also includes the salivary glands, mouth, esophagus, liver, pancreas, gallbladder, and rectum.

Gland: An organ that makes hormones, digestive juices, sweat, tears, saliva, milk or other bodily substances. Endocrine glands release the substances directly into the bloodstream. Exocrine glands release the substances into a duct or opening to the inside or outside of the body.

Grading: A system for classifying cancer cells in terms of how abnormal they appear when examined under a microscope. The objective of a grading system is to provide information about the probable growth rate of the tumor and its tendency to spread. The systems used to grade tumors vary with each type of cancer. Grading plays a role in treatment decisions.

Growth Factor: A substance made by the body that functions to regulate cell division and cell survival. Some growth factors are also produced in the laboratory and used in biological therapy.

Healing Touch: A type of CAM based on the belief that a vital energy flows through the human body. This energy is said to be balanced or made stronger by practitioners who pass their hands over a patient's body. Healing touch is being studied in patients receiving cancer treatments to find out if it can improve quality of life, boost the immune system or reduce side effects Also called therapeutic touch.

Homeopathy: A compendium of remedies based on the belief that natural substances, prepared in a special way and used in minute amounts, restore health. Often known as "like cures like," in order for a remedy to be effective it must cause in a healthy person the same symptoms being treated in the patient.

Hormone: Chemicals made by glands in the body. Hormones circulate in the bloodstream and control the actions of certain cells or organs. Some hormones, like estrogen, can also be made in the laboratory.

Immunocompromised: Having a weakened immune system caused by certain diseases or treatments.

Immunomodulation: Change in the body's immune system, caused by agents that activate or suppress its function.

Immunostimulant: A substance that increases the ability of the immune system to fight infection and disease.

Insulin: A hormone made by the islet cells of the pancreas. Insulin controls the amount of sugar in the blood by moving it into the cells, where it can be used by the body for energy.

Insulin Growth Factor (IGF): A protein made by the body that stimulates the growth of many types of cells. IGF is similar to insulin (a hormone made in the pancreas). There are two forms of IGF called IGF-1 and IGF-2. Higher than normal levels of IGF-1 may increase the risk of several types of cancer. IGF is a type of growth factor and a type of cytokine.

Islet Cell Carcinoma: A rare cancer that forms in the islets of Langerhans cells. Also called pancreatic endocrine cancer.

Islet of Langerhans Cell: A pancreatic cell that produces hormones (e.g., insulin and glucagon) that are secreted into the bloodstream. These hormones help control the level of glucose (sugar) in the blood. Also called endocrine pancreas cell and islet cell.

Jaundice: A condition in which the skin and the whites of the eyes become yellow, urine darkens, and the color of stool becomes lighter than normal. Jaundice occurs when the liver is not working properly or when a bile duct is blocked.

Killer T-Cell: A type of immune cell that can kill certain cells, including foreign cells, cancer cells, and cells infected with a virus. Killer T-cells can be separated from other blood cells, grown in the laboratory, and then given to a patient to kill cancer cells. A killer T-cell is a type of white blood cell and a type of lymphocyte.

Kras Gene: A gene that may cause cancer when it is mutated. The Kras gene makes the KRAS protein, which is involved in cell signaling pathways, cell growth, and apoptosis (cell death). Agents that block the activity of the mutated Kras gene or its protein may stop the growth of cancer.

Laparoscopy: A procedure that uses a laparoscope, inserted through the abdominal wall, to examine the inside of the abdomen. A laparoscope is a thin, tube-like instrument with a light and a lens for viewing. It may also have a tool to remove tissue to be checked under a microscope for signs of disease.

Late Stage Cancer: A term used to describe cancer that is far along in its growth, and has spread to the lymph nodes or other places in the body.

Latent: Describes a condition that is present but not active or causing symptoms.

Lesion: An area of abnormal tissue. A lesion may be benign (not cancer) or malignant (cancer).

Locally Advanced: If the cancer has not spread to distant organs but it still can't be completely removed with surgery, it is called locally advanced. Often the reason the cancer can't be removed is because too much of it is present in nearby blood vessels. Since the cancer cannot be removed entirely by surgery, it is also called unresectable. For these tumors, surgery would only be done to relieve symptoms or problems like a blocked bile duct or intestinal tract.

Lymph: The clear fluid that travels through the lymphatic system and carries cells that help fight infections and other diseases. Also called lymphatic fluid.

Lymph Node: A rounded mass of lymphatic tissue that is surrounded by a capsule of connective tissue. Lymph nodes filter lymph (lymphatic fluid), and they store lymphocytes (white blood cells). They are located along lymphatic vessels. Also called lymph gland.

Malignancy: A term for diseases in which abnormal cells divide without control and can invade nearby tissues. Malignant cells can also spread to other parts of the body through the blood and lymph systems. There are several main types of malignancy. Carcinoma is a malignancy that begins in the skin or in tissues that line or cover internal organs. Sarcoma is a malignancy that begins in bone, cartilage, fat, muscle, blood vessels, or other connective or supportive tissue. Leukemia is a malignancy that starts in blood-forming tissue such as the bone marrow, and causes large numbers of abnormal blood cells to be produced and enter the blood. Lymphoma and multiple myeloma are malignancies that begin in the cells of the immune system. Central nervous system cancers are malignancies that begin in the tissues of the brain and spinal cord.

Maximum Tolerated Dose: The highest dose of a drug or treatment that does not cause unacceptable side effects. The maximum tolerated dose is determined in clinical trials by testing increasing doses on different groups of people until the highest dose with acceptable side effects is found. Also called MTD.

Mesothelin: A protein found on the surface of certain types of normal cells and cancer cells. Mesothelin may help these cells stick together and send signals. A higher-than-normal amount of mesothelin is found on some cancer cells, including mesothelioma, pancreatic cancer, and ovarian cancer.

Metastasize: The spread of cancer from one organ or part of the body to another non-adjacent area. For instance, cancer cells can break away, leak, or spill from a primary tumor, enter lymphatic and blood vessels, circulate through the bloodstream, and be deposited within normal tissue elsewhere in the body.

Metronomic Dosing: The long-term, low-dose, frequent administration of chemotherapeutic drugs. Rather than directly killing cancer cells, it prevents blood-vessel formation by blocking endothelial-cell growth. It also has the benefit of reducing the severity of chemotherapy side effects.

Mindfulness Relaxation: A type of meditation based on the concept of being "mindful," or having increased awareness, of the present. It uses breathing methods, guided imagery, and other practices to relax the body and mind and help reduce stress.

Mitochondria: Small structures in a cell that are found in the cytoplasm (fluid that surrounds the cell nucleus). Mitochondria make most of the energy for the cell and have their own genetic material that is different from the genetic material found in the nucleus. Many diseases are caused by mutations (changes) in the DNA of mitochondria. Mitochondria are cell organelles.

Mutation: Any change in the DNA of a cell. Mutations may be caused by mistakes during cell division, or they may be caused by exposure to DNA-damaging agents in the environment. Mutations can be harmful, beneficial, or have no effect. If they occur in cells that make eggs or sperm, they can be inherited; if mutations occur in other types of cells, they are not inherited. Certain mutations may lead to cancer or other diseases.

Natural Killer Cell: A cell that can destroy another cell without prior sensitization to it. Natural killer (NK) cells are part of our first line of defense against cancer cells and virus-infected cells.

Needle Biopsy: The removal of tissue or fluid with a needle for examination under a microscope. When a wide needle is used, the procedure is called a core biopsy. When a thin needle is used, the procedure is called a fine-needle aspiration biopsy.

Neoplasm: An abnormal mass of tissue that results when cells divide more than they should or do not die when they should. Neoplasms may be benign (not cancer), or malignant (cancer). Also called tumor.

Occult Primary Tumor: Cancer in which the site of the primary (original) tumor cannot be found. Most metastases from occult primary tumors are found in the head and neck.

Oncologist: A doctor who specializes in treating cancer. Some oncologists specialize in a particular type of cancer treatment. For example, a chemotherapy oncologist specializes in treating cancer with chemotherapeutic drugs.

Oncology: The study of cancer.

Open Biopsy: A procedure in which a surgical incision is made through the skin to expose and remove tissues. The biopsy tissue is then examined under a microscope by a pathologist. An open biopsy may be done in the doctor's office or in the hospital, and may use local anesthesia or general anesthesia. A lumpectomy to remove a breast tumor is a type of open biopsy.

Organelle: Structures inside a cell, such as mitochondria, that perform a specific function.

Oxidation: A chemical reaction that takes place when a substance comes into contact with oxygen or another oxidizing substance. Examples of oxidation are rust and the brown color on a cut apple.

Oxidative Stress: A condition in which antioxidant levels are lower than normal. Antioxidant levels are usually measured in blood plasma.

Pallative Care: Care given to improve the quality of life of patients who have a serious or life-threatening disease. The goal of palliative care is to prevent or treat as early as possible the symptoms of a disease, side effects caused by treatment of a disease, and psychological, social, and spiritual problems related to a disease or its treatment.

Pancreatectomy: Surgery to remove all or part of the pancreas. In a total pancreatectomy, part of the stomach, part of the small intestine, the common bile duct, gallbladder, spleen, and nearby lymph nodes are also removed.

Pancreatitis: Inflammation of the pancreas. Chronic pancreatitis may cause diabetes and problems with digestion. Pain is the primary symptom.

Peritoneal Cavity: The space within the abdomen that contains the intestines, the stomach, and the liver. It is bound by thin membranes.

Primary Tumor: The original tumor.

Refractory Cancer: Cancer that does not respond to treatment. The cancer may be resistant at the beginning of treatment or it may become resistant during treatment. Also called resistant cancer.

Regression: A decrease in the size of a tumor or in the extent of cancer in the body.

Remission: A decrease in or disappearance of signs and symptoms of cancer. In partial remission, some, but not all, signs and symptoms of cancer have disappeared. In complete remission, all signs and symptoms of cancer have disappeared, although it is possible that cancer is still in the body.

Resectable: If the cancer is only in the pancreas (or has spread just beyond it) and the surgeon can remove the entire tumor, it is called resectable.

Signal Transduction: The process by which a cell responds to substances in its environment. The binding of a substance to a molecule on the surface of a cell causes signals to be passed from one molecule to another inside the cell. These signals can affect many functions of the cell, including cell division and cell death. Cells that have permanent changes in signal transduction molecules may develop into cancer.

Signaling Pathway: A group of molecules in a cell that work together to control one or more cell functions, such as cell division or cell death. After the first molecule in a pathway receives a signal, it activates another molecule. This process is repeated until the last molecule is activated and the task is completed. Abnormal activation of signaling pathways can lead to cancer, and drugs are being developed to block these pathways. This may help block cancer cell growth and kill cancer cells.

Sphincterotomy: A relatively new endoscopic technique developed to examine and treat abnormalities of the bile ducts, pancreas, and gallbladder.

Staging: Performing exams and tests to learn the extent of the cancer within the body, especially whether the disease has spread from the original site to other parts of the body. It is important to know the stage of the disease in order to plan the best treatment.

Terminal Disease: Disease that cannot be cured and will cause death.

Total Parenteral Nutrition: A form of nutrition that is delivered into a vein. Total parenteral nutrition does not use the digestive system. It may be given to people who are unable to absorb nutrients through the intestinal tract because of vomiting that won't stop, severe diarrhea or intestinal disease. It may also be given to those undergoing high-dose chemotherapy or radiation and bone marrow transplantation. It is possible to give all of the protein, calories, vitamins, and minerals a person needs using total parenteral nutrition.

Tumor: An abnormal mass of tissue that results when cells divide more than they should or do not die when they should. Tumors may be benign (not cancer), or malignant (cancer). Also called neoplasm.

Tumor Burden: Refers to the number of cancer cells, the size of a tumor, or the amount of cancer in the body. Also called tumor load.

Tumor Necrosis Factor: A protein made by white blood cells in response to an antigen (substance that causes the immune system to make a specific immune response) or infection. Tumor necrosis factor can also be made in the laboratory. It may boost a person's immune response, and also may cause necrosis (cell death) of some types of tumor cells. Tumor necrosis factor is being studied in the treatment of some types of cancer. It is a type of cytokine.

Ultrasound: A procedure in which high-energy sound waves are bounced off internal tissues or organs and make echoes. The echo patterns are shown on the screen of an ultrasound machine, forming a picture of body tissues called a sonogram.

Unresectable: See *Locally advanced.*

Video-Assisted Resection: Surgery that is aided by the use of a video camera that projects and enlarges the image on a television screen.

Whipple Procedure: A complex type of surgery used to treat pancreatic cancer. The head of the pancreas, the duodenum, a portion of the stomach, and other nearby tissues are removed.

White Blood Cell: A type of immune cell. Most white blood cells are made in the bone marrow and are found in the blood and lymph tissue. White blood cells help the body fight infections and diseases.

Selected References
by Chapter

CHAPTER 1

http://www.hmc.psu.edu/healthinfo/pq/pancreaticcancer.htm

Documents and Photographs Related to Japanese Relocation During World War II. National Archives. http://www.archives.gov/education/lessons/japanese-relocation

Randall V. Internment of Japanese Americans in Concentration Camps. University of Dayton. http://academic.udayton.edu/race/02rights/intern01.htm

Transcript of Executive Order 9066 by President Franklin Roosevelt, February 19, 1942. Available from OurDocuments.gov: http://www.ourdocuments.gov/doc.php?flash=true&doc=74

CHAPTER 2

Forst T. Molecular effects of C-Peptide in microvascular blood flow regulation. *Review of Diabetic Studies*. 6(3):159-167, 2009.

Iglesias García J. Endoscopic ultrasound in the diagnosis and staging of pancreatic cancer. *Revista Española de Enfermedades Digestivas*. 101(9):631-8, 2009.

New Blood Test for Detecting early Stage Pancreatic Cancer Presented at Cancer Conference. CNN Money. 21 Jan 2010.

Park SS. Diagnostic usefulness of PET/CT for pancreatic malignancy. *Korean Journal of Gastroenterology*. 54(4):235-242, 2009.

Stages of Pancreatic Cancer. National Cancer Institute. 2009.

Tortora GJ and Bryan Derrickson. Principles of Anatomy and Physiology. Wiley: New York. 942-944, 2008.

Touchefeu Y. Endoscopic ultrasound-guided fine-needle aspiration for the diagnosis of solid pancreatic masses: the impact on patient-management strategy. *Alimentary Pharmacology & Therapeutics*. 30(10):1070-1077, 2009.

van der Gaag NA. Preoperative biliary drainage for cancer of the head of the pancreas. *New England Journal of Medicine*. 2010 Jan 14;362(2):129-37.

Verspohl EJ. Muscarinic receptor subtypes in rat pancreatic islets: binding and functional studies. *European Journal of Pharmacology*. 178(3):303-311, 1990.

Wenner M. What makes pancreatic cancer so deadly? *Scientific American*. 24 Aug 2008.

Wong JC. Staging of pancreatic adenocarcinoma by imaging studies. *Clinical Gastroenterology and Hepatology*. 6(12):1301-1308, 2008.

Wong KK. Incremental Value of 111-In Pentetreotide SPECT/CT Fusion Imaging of Neuroendocrine Tumors. *Academic Radiology*. 2009 Dec 3. [Epub ahead of print]

CHAPTER 3

http://www.cancer.org/docroot/CRI/content/CRI_2_4_1X_What_are_the_key_statistics_for_pancreatic_cancer_34.asp

Aitken-Swan J. Reactions of Cancer Patients on Being Told Their Diagnosis. *British Medical Journal*. 1(5124): 779-780, 781-783, 1959.

Aoki C. Differences among Asian American ethnicities with hepatocelluar carcinoma in California. Abstract 123. Presented at the 2009 Gastrointestinal Cancers Symposium. 2009.

Chen JM. Loss of function, mutations in the cationic trypsinogen gene (PRSS1) may act as a protective factor against pancreatitis. *Molecular Genetics and Metabolism*. 79(1):67-70. 2003.

Chen MS. Jr. Cancer health disparities among Asian Americans: what we do and what we need to do. *Cancer*. 104(12 Suppl):2895-902, 2005.

Fleming JB. Influence of obesity on cancer-related outcomes after pancreatectomy to treat pancreatic adenocarcinoma. *Archives of Surgery*. 144(3):216-221. 2009.

Genkinger JM. Alcohol intake and pancreatic cancer risk: A pooled analysis of fourteen cohort studies. *Cancer Epidemiological Biomarkers & Prevention*. 18: 765-76. 2009.

Grocock CJ. The variable phenotype of the p.A16V mutation of cationic trypsinogen (PRSS1) in pancreatitis families. doi:10.1136/gut.2009.186817. 2009.

Horner MJ. SEER Cancer Statistics Review, 1975-2006. National Cancer Institute. Bethesda, MD, http://seer.cancer.gov/csr/1975_2006/, based on November 2008 SEER data submission, posted to the SEER Web site, 2009.

Huxley R. Type-II diabetes and pancreatic cancer: a meta-analysis of 36 studies. *British Journal of Cancer*. 92(11):2076-2083. 2005.

Jee SH. Fasting serum glucose level and cancer risk in Korean men and women. *Journal of the American Medical Association*. 293(2):194-202. 2005.

Johansen D. Different markers of alcohol consumption, smoking and body mass index in relation to risk of pancreatic cancer. A prospective cohort study within the Malmö Preventive Project. *Pancreatology*. 9(5):677-686. 2009.

Ji BT. Occupational Exposure to Pesticides and Pancreatic Cancer. 39;92-99. 2001.

Kernan GJ. Occupational risk factors for pancreatic cancer: a case-control study based on death certificates from 24 U.S. states. *American Journal of Industrial Medicine*. 36(2): 260-270. 1999.

Larsson SC. Consumption of sugar and sugar-sweetened foods and the risk of pancreatic cancer in a prospective study. *American Journal of Clinical Nutrition*. 84(5) 1171-1176. 2006.

Luo J. Obesity and risk of pancreatic cancer among postmenopausal women: the Women's Health Initiative (United States). *British Journal of Cancer*. 99: 527–531. 2008.

Michaud DS. Dietary sugar, glycemic load, and pancreatic cancer risk in a prospective study. *Journal of the National Cancer Institute*. 94(17):1293-300. 2002.

Ojajärvi A. Occupational exposures and pancreatic cancer: a meta-analysis. *Occupational and Environmental Medicine*. **57:**316-324. 2000.

Rasmussen A. Uptake of genetic testing and long-term tumor surveillance in von Hippel-Lindau disease. *BMC Medical Genetics.* 11(1):4. 2010.

Shacter E. Chronic inflammation and cancer. *Oncology.* 16(2):217-26, 229. 2002.

Song Z. Potential carcinogenic effects of cigarette smoke and Swedish moist snuff on pancreas: a study using a transgenic mouse model of chronic pancreatitis. *Laboratory Investigation.* 2010 Jan 11. [Epub ahead of print]

Tai MH. Cigarette smoke components inhibited intercellular communication and differentiation in human pancreatic ductal epithelial cells. *International Journal of Cancer.* 120(9):1855-1862. 2007.

Thiébaut ACM. Dietary Fatty Acids and Pancreatic Cancer in the NIH-AARP Diet and Health Study. *Journal of the National Cancer Institute.* 101(14):1001-1011. 2009.

Wasif Saif M. Impact of Ethnicity on Outcome in Pancreatic Carcinoma. *Journal of the Pancreas (Online).* 6(2):246-254. 2005.

CHAPTER 4

http://www.cancer.gov/cancertopics/chemo-side-effects

http://www.cancer.org

Bayraktar S. Recent developments in palliative chemotherapy for locally advanced and metastatic pancreas cancer. *World Journal of Gastroenterology.* 16(6):673-82. 2010.

Collins A. Diagnosis and management of pancreatic cancer. *Minerva Gastroenterologica Dietologica.* 55(4):445-54. 2009.

Dong K. Analysis of multiple factors of postsurgical gastroparesis syndrome after pancreaticoduodenectomy and cryotherapy for pancreatic cancer. *World Journal of Gastroenterology.* 10(16):2434-2438. 2004.

Fujino Y. Impact of gemcitabine on the survival of patients with stage IV pancreatic cancer. *Pancreas.* 34(3):335-339. 2007.

Lai EC. Measures to prevent pancreatic fistula after pancreatoduodenectomy: a comprehensive review. *Archives of Surgery.* 144(11):1074-1080. 2009.

Maruyama Y. Perioperative challenges associated with a pancreaticoduodenectomy and distal pancreatectomy for pancreatic cancer in patients with situs inversus totalis: report of two cases. *Surgery Today.* 40(1):79-82. 2010.

Nakeeb A. Surgical techniques for pancreatic cancer. *Minerva Chirurgica.* 59(2):151-163. 2004.

National Cancer Institute Fact Sheet 7.49, Targeted Cancer Therapies: Questions and Answers. http://www.cancer.gov/cancertopics/factsheet/Therapy/targeted

Okabayashi T. Long-term effects of multimodal treatment for patients with resectable carcinoma of the pancreas. *Oncology Reports.* 20(3):651-656. 2008.

Radiation Therapy and You: Support for People With Cancer. http://www.cancer.gov/cancertopics/radiation-therapy-and-you.

Royall D. Nutritional status and function in patients following Whipple procedure compared with controls. *Journal of the American College of Nutrition.* 15 (1):73-78. 1996.

Saruç M. Pancreatic cancer and glucose metabolism. *Turkish Journal of Gastroenterology.* 20(4):257-260. 2009.

Shibuya K. Phase II Study of Radiation Therapy Combined With Weekly Low-Dose Gemcitabine for Locally Advanced, Unresectable Pancreatic Cancer. *American Journal of Clinical Oncology.* 2010 Jan 8. [Epub ahead of print]

Spanknebel K. Advances in the surgical management of pancreatic cancer. *Cancer Journal.* 7(4):312-323. 2001.

Tien YW. Enteral nutrition and biliopancreatic diversion effectively minimize impacts of gastroparesis after pancreaticoduodenectomy. *Journal of Gastrointestinal Surgery.* 13(5):929-937. 2009.

Yang R. Survival effects of adjuvant chemoradiotherapy after resection for pancreatic carcinoma. *Archives of Surgery.* 145(1):49-56. 2010.

Zhongmin W. Clinical efficacy of CT-guided iodine-125 seed implantation therapy in patients with advanced pancreatic cancer. *European Radiology.* 2010 Jan 13. [Epub ahead of print]

CHAPTER 5

Bergers G. Combining antiangiogenic agents with metronomic chemotherapy enhances efficacy against late-stage pancreatic islet carcinomas in mice. *Cold Springs Harbor Symposia of Quantatative Biology.* 67:293-300. 2002.

Bocci G. Thrombospondin 1, a mediator of the antiangiogenic effects of low-dose metronomic chemotherapy. *Proceedings of the National Academy of Sciences USA.* 100: 12917–12922. 2003.

Carlson RH. Metronomic timing adds antiangiogenic punch. *Oncology Times.* 24(1): 32-24. 2002.

Chue BM. Five-year survival of metastatic pancreatic carcinoma: a study of courage and hope. *Gastrointestinal Cancer Research.* 3(5):208-211. 2009.

Hanahan D. Less is more, regularly: metronomic dosing of cytotoxic drugs can target tumor angiogenesis in mice. *Journal of Clinical Investigation.* 105(8):1045-1047. 2000.

Hoshino H. A long-term survival case of pancreatic cancer with hepatic metastasis after pancreaticoduodenectomy successfully treated by s-1 and gemcitabine combination chemotherapy. *Gan To Kagaku Ryoho.* 36(12):2419-2421. 2009.

Kim MP. Gemcitabine Resistance in Pancreatic Cancer: Picking the Key Players. *Clinical Cancer Research.* 14; 1284-1285. 2008.

Matsubara J. Survival prediction for pancreatic cancer patients receiving gemcitabine treatment. *Molecular & Cellular Proteomics.* 2010 Jan 8. [Epub ahead of print]

Petrangolini G. Combination of metronomic gimatecan and CpG-oligodeoxynucleotides against an orthotopic pancreatic cancer xenograft. *Cancer Biology & Therapy.* 7(4):596-601. 2008.

Pietras K. A multitargeted, metronomic, and maximum-tolerated dose "chemo-switch" regimen is antiangiogenic, producing objective responses and survival benefit in a mouse model of cancer. *Journal of Clinical Oncology.* 23(5):939-952. 2005.

Shaked Y. Optimal biologic dose of metronomic chemotherapy regimens is associated with maximum antiangiogenic activity. *Blood.* 106(9): 3058–3061. 2005.

Xie DR. Gemcitabine-based Cytotoxic Doublets Chemotherapy for Advanced Pancreatic Cancer: Updated Subgroup Meta-analyses of Overall Survival. *Japanese Journal of Clinical Oncology.* 2010 Feb 10. [Epub ahead of print]

CHAPTER 6

Albini A. Inhibition of Angiogenesis and Vascular Tumor Growth by Interferon-Producing Cells. *American Journal of Pathology.* 156:1381-1393. 2000.

Amara S. Oral glutamine for the prevention of chemotherapy-induced peripheral neuropathy. *Annals of Pharmacotherapy.* 42(10):1481-1485. 2008.

Anderson RA. Elevated intakes of supplemental chromium improve glucose and insulin variables in individuals with type 2 diabetes. *Diabetes.* 46(11):1786-1791. 1997.

Ang CD. Vitamin B for treating peripheral neuropathy. *Cochrane Database System Review.* (3):CD004573. 2008.

Bar-Sela G. Curcumin as an Anti-Cancer Agent: Review of the Gap between Basic and Clinical Applications. *Current Medicinal Chemistry.* 2009 Nov 24. [Epub ahead of print].

Bayram I. The use of a protein and energy dense eicosapentaenoic acid containing supplement for malignancy-related weight loss in children. *Pediatric Blood & Cancer.* 52(5):571-574. 2009.

Bennett P. Naturopathy Complements Chemo. *Alive: Canadian Journal of Health & Nutrition.* 234: 46. 2002.

Berrington de Gonzalez A. Pancreatic Cancer and Factors Associated with the Insulin Resistance Syndrome in the Korean Cancer Prevention Study. *Cancer Epidemiology, Biomarkers & Prevention.* 17; 359. 2008.

Block G. Vitamin C and cancer prevention: the epidemiologic evidence. *American Journal of Clinical Nutrition.* 53: 270S-282S. 1991.

Block KI. Impact of Antioxidant Supplementation on Chemotherapeutic Efficacy: A Systematic Review of the Evidence from Randomized Controlled Trials. *Cancer Treatment Reviews.* 33(5):407-418. 2007.

Bougnoux P. Improving outcome of chemotherapy of metastatic breast cancer by docosahexaenoic acid: a phase II trial. *British Journal of Cancer.* 101(12):1978-85. 2009.

Boukhettala N. A Diet Containing Whey Protein, Glutamine, and TGFbeta Modulates Gut Protein Metabolism During Chemotherapy-Induced Mucositis in Rats. *Digestive Diseases and Sciences.* 2009 Nov 13. [Epub ahead of print]

Bounous G. Whey protein concentrate (WPC) and glutathione modulation in cancer treatment. *Anticancer Research.* 20(6C):4785-4792. 2000.

Casado-Zapico S. Synergistic antitumor effect of melatonin with several chemotherapeutic drugs on human Ewing sarcoma cancer cells: potentiation of the extrinsic apoptotic pathway. *Journal of Pineal Research.* 48(1):72-80. 2010.

Cenacchi T. Cognitive decline in the elderly: a double-blind, placebo-controlled multicenter study on efficacy of phosphatidylserine administration. *Aging (Milano).* 5(2):123-133. 1993.

Conklin KA. Coenzyme q10 for prevention of anthracycline-induced cardiotoxicity. *Integrative Cancer Therapies.* 4(2):110-130. 2005.

Conklin KA. Dietary antioxidants during cancer chemotherapy: impact on chemotherapeutic effectiveness and development of side effects. *Nutritional Cancer.* 37(1):1-18. 2000.

Crew KD. Association between plasma 25-hydroxyvitamin D and breast cancer risk. *Cancer Prevention Research (Phila Pa).* 2(6):598-604. 2009.

Cruciani RA. Safety, tolerability and symptom outcomes associated with L-carnitine supplementation in patients with cancer, fatigue, and carnitine deficiency: a phase I/II study. *Journal of Pain Symptom Management.* 32(6):551-559. 2006.

D'Andrea GM. Use of antioxidants during chemotherapy and radiotherapy should be avoided. *CA: A Cancer Journal for Clinicians.* 55(5):319-321. 2005.

Danielczyk K. MT1 melatonin receptors and their role in the oncostatic action of melatonin. *Postępy higieny i medycyny doświadczalnej (Online).* 63:425-34. 2009.

DeVita DT. A History of Cancer Chemotherapy. *Cancer Research.* 68:8643. 2008.

Dubost J. Identification and quantification of L-ergothioneine, identification of selenoergothioneine and quantification of polyphenols in cultivated mushrooms. Presented at the American Chemical Society's Second International Congress on Antioxidant Methods. June 22-24, 2005.

Ebbing M. Cancer incidence and mortality after treatment with folic acid and vitamin B12. *Journal of the American Medical Association.* 302(19):2119-2126. 2009.

El-Shemy HA. Antitumor Properties and Modulation of Antioxidant Enzymes' Activity by Aloe vera Leaf Active Principles Isolated by Supercritical Carbon Dioxide Extraction. *Current Medicinal Chemistry.* 2009 Nov 24. [Epub ahead of print]

Fife J. Folic Acid Supplementation and Colorectal Cancer Risk; A Meta-analysis. Colorectal Disease. 2009 Oct 27. [Epub ahead of print]

Fletcher RH. Vitamins for Chronic Disease Prevention in Adults: Scientific Review. *Journal of the American Medical Association.* 287:3116-3126. 2002.

Gao Y. Effects of ganopoly (a Ganoderma lucidum polysaccharide extract) on the immune functions in advanced-stage cancer patients. *Immunological Investigations.* 32(3):201-215. 2003.

Garland CF. The Role of Vitamin D in Cancer Prevention. *American Journal of Public Health.* 10.2105/AJPH.2004.045260. 2006.

Girón RA. Dehydroepiandrosterone inhibits the proliferation and induces the death of HPV-positive and HPV-negative cervical cancer cells through an androgen- and estrogen-receptor independent mechanism. *FEBS Journal.* 276(19):5598-609. 2009.

Glycyrrhiza glabra – monograph. *Alternative Medicine Review.* 10:230-237. 2005.

Gröber U. Vitamin C in complementary oncology--update 2009. *Med Monatsschr Pharm.* 32(7):263-267. 2009.

Habermann N. Fish fatty acids alter markers of apoptosis in colorectal adenoma and adenocarcinoma cell lines but fish consumption has no impact on apoptosis-induction ex vivo. *Apoptosis.* 2010 Jan 28. [Epub ahead of print]

Heaney ML. Vitamin C Antagonizes the Cytotoxic Effects of Antineoplastic Drugs. *Cancer Research.* 68: 8031-8038. 2008.

Ishikawa H. Aged garlic extract prevents a decline of NK cell number and activity in patients with advanced cancer. *Journal of Nutrition.* 136(3 Suppl):816S-820S. 2006.

Johnston CJ. Vitamin C elevates red blood cell glutathione in healthy adults. *American Journal of Clinical Nutrition.* 58:103-105. 1993.

Joseph EK. Oxaliplatin acts on IB4-positive nociceptors to induce an oxidative stress-dependent acute painful peripheral neuropathy. *Pain.* 9(5):463-472. 2008.

Jung HJ. Evaluation of anti-angiogenic, anti-inflammatory and antinociceptive activity of coenzyme Q(10) in experimental animals. *Journal of Pharmacy and Pharmacology.* 61(10):1391-1395. 2009.

Kodama N. Can maitake MD-fraction aid cancer patients? *Alternative Medicine Review.* 7(3):236-239. 2002.

Konno S. A possible hypoglycaemic effect of maitake mushroom on Type 2 diabetic patients. *Diabetic Medicine*. 18:1010. 2001.

Ladas EJ. A Randomized, Controlled, Double-Blind, Pilot Study of Milk Thistle for the Treatment of Hepatotoxicity in Childhood Acute Lymphoblastic Leukemia (ALL). *Cancer*. 116(2):506-513. 2010.

Larsson SC. Folate intake and pancreatic cancer incidence: a prospective study of Swedish women and men. *Journal of the National Cancer Institute*. 98(6): 407-413. 2006.

Levine ME. Protein and ginger for the treatment of chemotherapy-induced delayed nausea. *Journal of Alternative and Complementary Medicine*. 14(5):545-551. 2008.

Li Y. Clinical trial: prophylactic intravenous alanyl-glutamine reduces the severity of gastrointestinal toxicity induced by chemotherapy--a randomized crossover study. *Alimentary Pharmacology & Therapeutics*. 30(5):452-458. 2009.

Marchionatti AM. Antiproliferative action of menadione and 1,25(OH)2D3 on breast cancer cells. *Journal of Steroid Biochemistry and Molecular Biology*. 113(3-5):227-32. 2009.

McKay DL. The effects of a multivitamin/mineral supplement on micronutrient status, antioxidant capacity and cytokin production in healthy older adults consuming a fortified diet. *Journal of the American College of Nutrition*. 19:613-621. 2000.

Ndhlala AR. Antimicrobial, anti-inflammatory and mutagenic investigation of the South African tree aloe (Aloe barbcrae). *Journal of Ethnopharmacology*. 124(3):404-408. 2009.

Pan L. Vitamin D stimulates apoptosis in gastric cancer cells in synergy with trichostatin A /sodium butyrate-induced and 5-aza-2'-deoxycytidine-induced PTEN upregulation. *FEBS Journal*. 277(4):989-99. 2010.

Poeggeler B. Melatonin, aging, and age-related diseases: perspectives for prevention, intervention, and therapy. *Endocrine*. 27:201-212. 2005.

Prieto-Hontoria PL. Lipoic acid prevents body weight gain induced by a high fat diet in rats: effects on intestinal sugar transport. *Journal of Physiology & Biochemistry*. 65(1):43-50. 2009.

Ravindran J. Curcumin and cancer cells: how many ways can curry kill tumor cells selectively? *The AAPS Journal*. 11(3):495-510. 2009.

Sergio GC. Activated charcoal to prevent irinotecan-induced diarrhea in children. *Pediatric Blood & Cancer*. 51(1):49-52. 2008.

Shen J. Potentiation of intestinal immunity by micellary mushroom extracts. *Biomedical Research*. 28(2):.71-77. 2007.

Singhal S. Thalidomide in cancer. *Biomedicine & Pharmacotherapy*. 56(1):4-12. 2002.

Somboonwong J. Therapeutic effects of Aloe vera on cutaneous microcirculation and wound healing in second degree burn model in rats. *Journal of the Medical Association of Thailand*. 83(4):417-425. 2000.

Takemura Y. High dose of ascorbic acid induces cell death in mesothelioma cells. *Biochemical and Biophysical Research Communications*. 2010 Feb 19. [Epub ahead of print]

Tufekci O. Evaluation of the effect of acetyl L-carnitine on experimental cisplatin nephrotoxicity. *Chemotherapy*. 55(6):451-459. 2009.

Vallianou N. Alpha-lipoic Acid and diabetic neuropathy. *Review of Diabetic Studies*. 6(4):230-236. 2009.

Venkataramanan R. Milk thistle, a herbal supplement, decreases the activity of CYP3A4 and uridine diphosphoglucoronosyl transferase in human hepatocyte cultures. *Drug Metabolism and Disposition*. 28:1270-1273. 2000.

Villegas I. New Mechanisms and therapeutic potential of curcumin for colorectal cancer. *Molecular Nutrition and Food Research*. 52(9):1040-1061. 2008.

Wang BJ. Free radical scavenging and apoptotic effects of Cordyceps sinensis fractionated by supercritical carbon dioxide. Food and Chemical Toxicology. 43:543-552. 2005.

Wang CZ. Effects of ganoderma lucidum extract on chemotherapy-induced nausea and vomiting in a rat model. *American Journal of Chinese Medicine*. 33(5):807-815. 2005.

Wang Y. Alpha-Lipoic acid increases energy expenditure by enhancing adenosine monophosphate-activated protein kinase-peroxisome proliferator-activated receptor-gamma coactivator-1alpha signaling in the skeletal muscle of aged mice. *Metabolism*. 2009 Dec 14. [Epub ahead of print]

Wang Y. Synthesis and preliminary antitumor activity evaluation of a DHA and doxorubicin conjugate. *Bioorganic & Medicinal Chemistry Letters*. 16(11):2974-2977. 2006.

Witschi A. The systemic availability of oral glutathione. *European Journal of Clinical Pharmacology*. 43(6):667-669. 1992.

White B. "Ginger: An Overview." *American Family Physician*. 75:1689-1691. 2007.

Xie H. Role of copper in angiogenesis and its medicinal implications. *Current Medicinal Chemistry*. 16(10):1304-1314. 2009.

Yance DR Jr. Targeting angiogenesis with integrative cancer therapies. *Integrative Cancer Therapies*. 5(1):9-29. 2006.

Zavorsky GS. An open-label dose-response study of lymphocyte glutathione levels in healthy men and women receiving pressurized whey protein isolate supplements. *International Journal of Food Sciences and Nutrition*. 58(6):429-36. 2007.

Zhou DH. Effect of Jinshuibao capsule on the immunological function of 36 patients with advanced cancer. *Zhongguo Zhong Xi Yi Jie He Za Zhi*. 15(8):476-478. 1995.

Zick SM. Phase II trial of encapsulated ginger as a treatment for chemotherapy-induced nausea and vomiting. *Supportive Care in Cancer*. 17(5):563-572. 2009.

CHAPTER 7

Asami DK. Comparison of the total phenolic and ascorbic acid content of freeze-dried and air-dried marionberry, strawberry, and corn grown using conventional, organic, and sustainable agricultural practices. *Journal of Agricultural and Food Chemistry*. 51:1237-1241. 2003.

Burros M. Is Organic Food Provably Better? *New York Times*. 16 July 2003.

Cancer: Diet and Physical Activity's Impact. Global Strategy on Diet, Physical Activity, and Health. World Health Organization. Available at www.who.int/dietphysicalactivity/publications/facts/cancer/en/

Carbonaro M. Modulation of antioxidant compounds in organic vs conventional fruit (peach, Prunus persica L., and pear, Pyrus communis L.). *Journal of Agricultural and Food Chemistry*. 50:5458-5462. 2002.

Flegal KM. Prevalence and trends in obesity among U.S. adults 1999-2008. *Journal of the American Medical Association*. 303(3):235-241. 2010.

Giovannucci E. Nutritional predictors of insulin-like growth factor I and their relationships to cancer in men. Cancer Epidemiology, Biomarkers and Prevention. 12:84-89. 2003

Jee SH. Fasting serum glucose level and cancer risk in Korean men and women. *Journal of the American Medical Association.* 293(2):194-202. 2005.

Kim J. Gastric cancer and salt preference: a population-based cohort study in Korea. *American Journal of Clinical Nutrition.* doi:10.3945/ajcn.2009.28732. 2010.

Lam TK. Cruciferous vegetable consumption and lung cancer risk: a systematic review. *Cancer Epidemiology, Biomarkers and Prevention.* 18:184-195. 2009.

Michaud DS. Dietary sugar, glycemic load, and pancreatic cancer risk in a prospective study. *Journal of the National Cancer Institute.* 94:1293-1300. 2002.

Nielsen SJ. Patterns and trends in food portion sizes, 1977-1998. *Journal of the American Medial Association.* 289(4):450-453. 2003.

Obesity and Other Diet- and Inactivity-Related Disease: National Impact, Costs, and Solutions. National Alliance for Nutrition and Activity (NANA). 2003.

Rolls BJ. Portion size of food affects energy intake in normal-weight and overweight men and women. *American Journal of Clinical Nutrition.* 76:1207-1213. 2002.

Shin A. Dietary intake of calcium, fiber and other micronutrients in relation to colorectal cancer risk: Results from the Shanghai Women's Health Study. *International Journal of Cancer.* 119:2938-2942. 2006.

Tsugane S. Salt and salted food intake and subsequent risk of gastric cancer among middle-aged Japanese men and women. *British Journal of Cancer.* 90(1):128-34. 2004.

Wansink B. Ice Cream Illusions: Bowls, spoons, and self-serve portion sizes. *American Journal of Preventive Medicine.* 31(3): 240-243. 2006.

Worthington V. Nutritional quality of organic versus conventional fruits, vegetables and grains. *Journal of Alternative and Complementary Medicine.* 7:161-173. 2001.

CHAPTER 8

Bao T. Use of acupuncture in the control of chemotherapy-induced nausea and vomiting. *Journal of the National Comprehensive Cancer Network.* 7(5):606-612. 2009.

Cerrone R. Efficacy of HT 7 point acupressure stimulation in the treatment of insomnia in cancer patients and in patients suffering from disorders other than cancer. *Minerva Medica.* 99(6):535-537. 2008.

Chen ZJ. Advances of clinical study on acupuncture and moxibustion for treatment of cancer pain. *Zhongguo Zhen Jiu.* 28(5):392-394. 2008.

Chen ZJ. Observation on the therapeutic effect of acupuncture at pain points on cancer pain. *Zhongguo Zhen Jiu.* 28(4):251-253. 2008.

Dibble SL. Acupressure for nausea: results of a pilot study. Oncology Nursing Forum. 27(1):41-47. 2000.

Gao SZ. Study on standardization of cupping technique: elucidation on the establishment of the National Standard Standardized Manipulation of Acupuncture and Moxibustion, Part V, Cupping. *Zhongguo Zhen Jiu.* 30(2):157-159. 2010.

Jeong HJ. Regulatory effect of cytokine production in asthma patients by SOOJI CHIM (Koryo Hand Acupuncture Therapy). *Immunopharmacology and Immunotoxicology.* 24(2):265-274. 2002.

Molassiotis A. The management of cancer-related fatigue after chemotherapy with acupuncture and acupressure: a randomised controlled trial. *Complementary Therapies in Medicine.* 15(4):228-237. 2007.

Roscoe JA. Acupressure bands are effective in reducing radiation therapy-related nausea. *Journal of Pain and Symptom Management.* 38(3):381-389. 2009.

Sima L. Therapeutic effect of acupuncture on cisplatin-induced nausea and vomiting. *Zhongguo Zhen Jiu.* 29(1):3-6. 2009.

Walker EM. Acupuncture versus venlafaxine for the management of vasomotor symptoms in patients with hormone receptor-positive breast cancer: a randomized controlled trial. *Journal of Clinical Oncology.* 28(4):634-640. 2010.

Wu P. Effects of moxa-cone moxibustion at Guanyuan on erythrocytic immunity and its regulative function in tumor-bearing mice. *Journal of Traditional Chinese Medicine.* 21(1):68-71. 2001.

Zhang T. Clinical research on nourishing yin and unblocking meridians recipe combined with opioid analgesics in cancer pain management. *Chinese Journal of Integrative Medicine.* 12(3):180-184. 2006.

Zhao CL. Effect of acupuncture on the activity of the peripheral blood T lymphocyte subsets and NK cells in patients with colorectal cancer liver metastasis. *Zhongguo Zhen Jiu.* 30(1):10-12. 2010.

CHAPTER 9

Adamsen L. Effect of a multimodal high intensity exercise intervention in cancer patients undergoing chemotherapy: randomized controlled trial. *British Medical Journal.* 339:b3410, doi: 10.1136/bmj.b3410. 2009.

Bennett MP. The effect of mirthful laughter on stress and natural killer cell activity. *Alternative Therapies in Health and Medicine.* 9: 38-45. 2003.

Bhattacharya S. Improvement in oxidative status with yogic breathing in young healthy males. *Indian Journal of Physiology and Pharmacology.* 46: 349-354. 2002.

Bränström R. Self-report Mindfulness as a Mediator of Psychological Well-being in a Stress Reduction Intervention for Cancer Patients-A Randomized Study. *Annals of Behavioral Medicine.* 2010 Feb 23. [Epub ahead of print]

Carlson LE. Mindfulness-based stress reduction in relation to quality of life, mood, symptoms of stress and levels of cortisol, dehydropiandrosterone sulfate (DHEAS) and melatonin in breast and prostate cancer outpatients. *Psychoneuroendocrinology.* 29:448-474. 2004.

Coker KH. Meditation and prostate cancer: integrating a mind/body intervention with traditional therapies. *Seminars in Urologic Oncology.* 17(2):111-118. 1999.

Foley E. Mindfulness-based cognitive therapy for individuals whose lives have been affected by cancer: a randomized controlled trial. *Journal of Consulting and Clinical Psychology.* 78(1):72-9. 2010.

Garssen B. On the role of immunological factors as mediators between psychosocial factors and cancer progression. *Psychiatry Research.* 85: 51-61. 1999.

Glaser R. Stress depresses interferon production by leukocytes concomitant with a decrease in natural killer cell activity. *Behavioral Neuroscience.* 100:675-678. 1986.

Halstead MT. Restoring the spirit at the end of life: music as an intervention for oncology nurses. *Clinical Journal of Oncology Nursing.* 6(6):332-336. 2002.

Infante JR. Catecholamine levels in practitioners of transcendental meditation technique. *Physiology & Behavior.* 72: 141-146. 2001.

Kiecolt-Glaser JK. Marital conflict in older adults: endocrinological and immuno-logical correlates. *Psychosomatic Medicine.* 59:350-351. 1997.

Kiecolt-Glaser JK. Negative behavior during marital conflict is associated with immunological down-regulation. *Psychosomatic Medicine.* 55:410-412. 1993.

Kiecolt-Glaser JK. Slowing of wound healing by psychological stress. *Lancet.* 346:1194-1196. 1995.

Kiecolt-Glaser JK. Distress and DNA repair in human lymphocytes. *Journal of Behavioral Medicine.* 8:311-320. 1985.

Kuchinski AM. Treatment-related fatigue and exercise in patients with cancer: a systematic review. *Medsurg Nursing.* 18(3):174-180. 2009.

Lazar SW. Functional brain mapping of the relaxation response and meditation. *Neuroreport.* 11: 1581-1585. 2000.

Moss M. Aromas of rosemary and lavender essential oils differentially affect cogni-tion and mood in healthy adults. *International Journal of Neuroscience.* 13:15-38. 2003.

O'Rorke MA. Can physical activity modulate pancreatic cancer risk? A systematic review and meta-analysis. *International Journal of Cancer.* 2009 Oct 23. [Epub ahead of print].

Resistance Training Improves Quality of Life in Older Cancer Survivors. *Medical News Today.* 29 May 2008.

Schlebusch KP. Biophotonics in the Infrared Spectral Range Reveal Acupuncture Meridian Structure of the Body. *The Journal of Alternative and Complementary Medicine.* 11(1): 171-173. 2005.

Schwartz AL. Effects of a 12-month randomized controlled trial of aerobic or resis-tence exercise during and following cancer treatment in women. *The Physician and Sportsmedicine.* 37(3):62-67. 2009.

Solberg EE. The effects of long meditation on plasma melatonin and blood sero-tonin. *Medical Science Monitor.* 10:CR96-101. 2004.

Speca M. A randomized wait-list control clinical trial: the effect of a mindfulness meditation-based stress reduction program on mood and symptoms of stress in cancer outpatients. *Psychosomatic Medicine.* 62:613-622. 2000.

Spence RR. Exercise and cancer rehabilitation: a systematic review. *Cancer Treatment Reviews.* 36(2):185-194. 2010.

CHAPTER 10

Carpenter K. Spirituality: a dimension of holistic critical care nursing. *Dimensions of Critical Care Nursing.* 27(1):16-20. 2008.

De Ridder D. Psychological adjustment to chronic disease. *The Lancet.* 372: 246-255. 2008.

Johnson ME. Centering prayer for women receiving chemotherapy for recurrent ovarian cancer: a pilot study. *Oncology Nursing Forum.* 36(4):421-428. 2009.

Jouret J. The power of positive thinking. *Lancet Oncology.* 11(3):230. 2010.

Meyers, S. Use of neurotransmitter precursors for treatment of depression. *Alternative Medicine Review.* 5:64-71. 2000.

Weihs KL. Negative affectivity, restriction of emotions, and site of metastases predict mortality in recurrent breast cancer. *Journal of Psychosomatic Research.* 49(1):59-68. 2000.

CHAPTER 11

Hodges LJ. Fear of recurrence and psychological distress in head and neck cancer patients and their carers. *Psychooncology*. 18(8):841-848. 2009.

Kenne Sarenmalm E. Experience and predictors of symptoms, distress and health-related quality of life over time in postmenopausal women with recurrent breast cancer. *Psychooncology*. 17(5):497-505. 2008.

Vivar CG. The psychosocial impact of recurrence on cancer survivors and family members: a narrative review. *Journal of Advanced Nursing*. 65(4):724-736. 2009.

Yang HC. Surviving recurrence: psychological and quality-of-life recovery. *Cancer*. 112(5):1178-1187. 2008.

CHAPTER 12

Fitzell A. Application of a stress and coping model to positive and negative adjustment outcomes in colorectal cancer caregiving. *Psychooncology*. 2009 Dec. 16. [Epub ahead of print]

Gysels MH. Caring for a person in advanced illness and suffering from breathlessness at home: threats and resources. *Palliative Support Care*. 7(2): 153-162. 2009.

H.R. 3248: Lifespan Respite Care Act of 2006. U.S. House of Representatives. Available at www.govtrack.us/congress/bill.xpd?bill=h109-3248.

Pariante CM. Chronic caregiving stress alters peripheral blood immune parameters: the role of age and severity of stress. *Psychotherapy and Psychosomatics*. 66(4): 199-207. 1997.

Prigerson HG. The Stressful Caregiving Adult Reactions to Experiences of Dying (SCARED) Scale: a measure for assessing caregiver exposure to distress in terminal care. *American Journal of Geriatric Psychiatry*. 11(3):309-319. 2003.

Rohleder N. Biologic cost of caring for a cancer patient: dysregulation of pro- and anti-inflammatory signaling pathways. *Journal of Clinical Oncology*. 27(18): 2909-2915. 2009.

Index

A

Abraxane, 123
Acetyl-l-carnitine, 74–75
Acupressure, 119
Acupuncture
    ailments treated by, 119
    benefits of, 120–24, 127–28
    initial visit for, 128–29
    meridians and, 118
    pain and, 121
    patient's attitude toward, 129
    safety of, 121
    types of, 118–20, 127
Adrenal glands, 133
Adrenaline, 133
Adriamycin, 96
African Americans, 26
Age, 20–21, 26
AGE (aged garlic extract), 75
Alcohol, 28
Aloe vera, 75–76
Alpha lipoic acid, 76
Amylase, 11, 18

Anemia, 54–55
Anger, 137, 151–53, 163
Angiography, 15–16
Antidepressants, 150–51
Antioxidants, 94, 96–97, 110–11
Anxiety, 137
Apoptosis, 18
Appetite, loss of, 8
Aromatherapy, 135–36, 137
Asthma, 134
Attitude, importance of, 34, 48, 72,
    129, 154–55
Avastin, 97

B

Beta carotene, 97
Bilirubin, 8, 12
Biofeedback, 136, 138
Bioflavonoids, 111
Biopsies, 16–17
Bloating, 8
Blood sugar levels, 8, 29
Blood tests, 12–13
Brachytherapy, 39

Breast cancer

   chemotherapy and, 52, 58, 63, 65,
      67, 78, 79, 119

   medicinal mushrooms and, 82, 83

   stress and, 135, 150

   vitamin D and, 89

Breathwork, 138

Bunch, Darin, 117–18, 125–30

C

CA 19-9, 12

Calcium, 87, 99

Cancer. *See also* Cancer treatment;
   Pancreatic cancer; Tests

   age and, 20–21

   causes of, 31

   coping with, 152–53

   diet and, 28–29, 100, 101–2, 104,
      108–15

   effects of, on family, 19, 33–34,
      42–43

   family history and, 26–27

   life before, 1–8

   reaction to diagnosis of, xvi–xvii,
      19, 149–50

   as reaffirmation of life, xvi, xviii,
      31–33

   recurrence of, 159–64, 165

   resources for, 183, 185–86

   spread of, 21–22

   stages of, 21, 22

Cancer treatment. *See also individual
   therapies*

   attitude and, 48

   conventional, 35–48

   failure of, 164–65

   future for, 72

   palliative, 165

Canned foods, 104

Carboplatin, 123

Caregivers

   advice for, 174–81

   breaks for, 179

   burnout of, 170–72

   emotions and, 178–79

   financial support for, 172

   importance of, 167–68

   number of, 168

   resources for, 183–84, 185

   rewards for, 181

   tasks performed by, 168, 169–71,
      172–75

Carotenes, 111

CEA (carcinoembryonic antigen), 12

Charcoal, activated, 75

"Chemo brain," 55, 86

Chemotherapy

   acupuncture and, 120–24, 127–28

   administering, 38

   antioxidants and, 94, 96–97

   benefits of, 36

   choosing oncologist for, 50–51

   combination, 35–36, 68–69

   definition of, 35

   eating problems and, 114, 116

   fear of, 62

   frequency and duration of, 37

   herbs and, 95

   maintaining strength during, 114

   metronomic vs. conventional,
      51–54, 58–59, 60, 62, 65–68, 73

   origins of, 61

   preparing for, 59–61

   preventing infections after, 84–85

   process of, 36–37

   side effects of, 37, 54–58, 63, 64,
      69–70, 73–91, 122–24

Chromium, 76

Chue, Ben, 50–54, 58–59, 62–63, 65–72, 117

Cisplatin, 75, 123, 161

Coenzyme Q10, 76

Coffee, 28

Colon cancer, 63, 65, 66, 72, 75, 77, 78, 82, 88, 89, 97

Confidence, 137

Control, 162

Cookbooks, 184

Cooking, 103. *See also* Diet

Coping strategies, 152–53, 164

Copper, 97

Cordyceps, 82

Cortisol, 133, 134

Courage, 156–57

CPT-11, 75, 161

CT (computed tomography) scan, 9–10, 11, 13–14

Cupping, 118–19

Curcumin, 77

D

Depression, 137, 150–51, 171–72

DGL (deglycyrrhizinated licorice), 78

DHA (docosahexaenoic acid), 78

DHEA (dehydroepiandrosterone), 77

Diabetes, 8, 26, 76, 101, 133

Diarrhea, 56, 75, 80, 116

Diet. *See also* Food

anticancer, 108–13, 115

for cancer patients, 108

as risk factor for cancer, 28–29, 100, 101–2, 104

standard American, 25, 99–100, 102, 104

Dishes, 107

Distress, 163

Docetaxel, 123

Doxorubicin, 74

E

Ear, acupuncture points on, 121

Eating problems, 114, 116

Edema, 55

Electroacupuncture (EA) machines, 120

Ellagic acid, 97

Emotions. *See also individual emotions*

aromatherapy and, 137

caregiving and, 178–79

dealing with, 154–55

expressing, 152

Enzyme levels, 11

EPA (eicosapentaenoic acid), 78

Epilepsy, 134

Epinephrine, 133

ERCP (endoscopic retrograde cholangiopancreatography), 10–11, 15

Essential oils, 135–36, 137

Estate planning, 174

Ethnicity, 26

Exercise, 29, 144–47

F

Faith, 153, 155–58

Family history, 26–27

Fat, 28, 101–2, 109

Fatigue, 122, 137, 163

Fear, 137

Fiber, 109–10

Fight-or-flight response, 133–34

Fish oil, 78, 95

Fistula, pancreatic, 40

5-fluorouracil, 63

Folic acid, 78–79

Food
    canned, 104
    fast, 107
    healthy vs. unhealthy, 112–13
    organic, 105–7
    portion sizes for, 106, 107
    processed, 104
Free radicals, 94, 96

G

Garlic extract, aged, 75
Gastroparesis, 40–41, 45
Gemcitabine, 36, 50, 63
Gemzar. *See* Gemcitabine
Genetics, 26–27
Ginger, 79
Glucagon, 17–18
Glutamine, 80–81
Glutathione, 81–82, 97
Glycemic index, 100, 101
Glycemic load, 101
Grief, 137
GTF (glucose tolerance factor), 76

H

Hair loss, 55–56
Happiness, 137
Health insurance, 173
Helicobacter pylori, 27
Herceptin, 65, 67
Hope, 152
Hypothalamus, 133

I

Immunity, boosting, 124
Imunosuppression, 56
Infections, preventing, 84–85
Insecurity, 137
Insomnia, 83, 171

Insulin, 17–18
Integrative medicine
    physicians' attitudes toward, xvii–xviii
    resources for, 187
Interferon, 69, 124
Irritability, 137
Islet cell cancers, 18
Islets of Langerhans, 18
Itching, 8

J

Jaundice, 8, 12

K

KRAS gene, 28

L

Lambright, Jim, 46–47
Laughter, 34, 138–39, 170
Legal issues, 173–74
Leucovorin, 63
Licorice. *See* DGL
Lifespan Respite Care Act, 172
Lipase, 11, 18
Liver cancer, 24, 82
Loneliness, 137
Love, 34
Lung cancer, 58, 66, 72, 82, 83, 110
Lymphoma, 61, 65, 67, 111

M

Magnesium, 99
Maitake, 82
Massage, 139
Meat
    cooking methods for, 102
    fats in, 28, 101–2
    processed, 102

Medications, managing, 80–81, 169. *See also individual medications*

Medicine, Eastern vs. Western, 129–30

Meditation, 139–40, 142

Melanoma, 83

Melatonin, 83

Memory, 137

MEN1 gene, 27

Meridians, 118

Metabolic syndrome, 76

Metastasis, 22

Milk thistle, 95

Mind-body therapies, 131, 189. *See also individual therapies*

Mindfulness, 139-140, 184

Mortality, coming to terms with, 153

Mouth sores, 114, 116

Moxibustion, 118

MRI (magnetic resonance imaging), 14

MTD (maximum tolerated dose), 54

Multivitamins, 83–86

Mushrooms, 82–83

Music therapy, 132

N

Naturopathic oncology, 90–93, 95

Nausea, 8, 56, 64, 79, 80, 116, 121

Needling, 118

Neuropathy, peripheral, 57, 70, 76, 122–24, 127–28

NF1 gene, 27

NK cells, 134

O

Obesity, 29–30, 104, 106

Occupational exposure, 30

OctreoScan, 14

Oils
    cooking, 109
    essential, 135–36, 137

Omega-3 fatty acids, 78, 110

Oncologists
    choosing, 50–51, 93
    initial appointment with, 70 71

Optimism, 152

Organic foods, 105–7

Ovarian cancer, 58, 89

Oxaliplatin, 63, 75, 123

P

Paclitaxel, 63, 74, 123

PAHs (polycyclic aromatic hydrocarbons), 30

Pain
    abdominal, 7
    reducing, 121 22, 120, 135

PAM4, 13

Pancreas
    functions of, 17–18
    size and shape of, 17
    structure of, 18

Pancreatectomy
    distal, 39–40
    total, 39

Pancreatic acini, 18

Pancreatic cancer
    causes of, 23–25, 31
    diagnosing, 12–17
    diet and, 100, 101–2
    effects of, 20
    endocrine, 18, 24
    exocrine, 18, 24
    metastatic, 22
    origins of, 18
    risk factors for, 12, 26–31

spread of, 18

stages of, 21, 22

survival rate for, 23, 24

symptoms of, 7–8

Pancreatitis

chronic, 27, 41

definition of, 11

Panic, 137

Pasteurization, 104

Patient advocates

caregivers as, 169

importance of, 71–72

resources for, 189–90

Pesticides, 30, 104

PET (positron emission tomography) scan, 14–15

Phosphatidylserine (PS), 86

Physical exams, 12

Plate size, 107

Portion sizes, 106, 107

Potassium, 99

Prayer, 141, 158

Present, living in, 32

Processed foods, 104

Prostate cancer, 77, 83, 110

Protein, 108, 109, 112–13

PRSS1 gene, 27

Q

Qi, 118, 119, 142

Quercetin, 86–87

R

Radiation therapy, 37, 39

Reilly, Paul, 73, 90–95, 104, 108, 110, 115

Reishi, 83

Relaxation exercises, 141

Research, database of, 190

Rituxan, 65

Rosenbaum, Ernest, 152

S

SAD (standard American diet), 25, 99–100, 102, 104

Salt, 101

Selenium, 96, 97, 111

Self-doubt, 163

Self-esteem, 153

Setbacks, dealing with, 159–65

Shiitake, 83

Smoking, 30

Smoothies, 110

Social Security, 173

Sodas, 100

Sodium, 101

Somatostatin receptor scintigraphy, 14

Spirituality, 153, 155–58

Sports, 132

Stomach cancer, 24, 66, 101, 111

Stool, changes in, 8

Stress

acupuncture and, 128

cancer and, 132, 134

effects of, 133–34

reducing, 135–44, 170

Sugar, 28–29, 101, 109

Supplements. *See also individual supplements*

buying, 87

managing, 80–81, 169

multivitamin, 83–86

resources for, 187–88

storing, 87

taking, 87, 93–94

Support groups, 152, 191

Surgery
  choosing surgeon for, 40–41
  recovery from, 44–48
  types of, 39–41

T

Tai chi, 142
Tea, green, 111
Tests
  angiography, 15–16
  biopsies, 16–17
  blood, 12–13
  CT scan, 9–10, 11, 13–14
  ERCP, 10, 11, 15
  MRI, 14
  OctreoScan, 14
  PET scan, 14–15
  somatostatin receptor scintigraphy, 14
  ultrasound, 15
Thalidomide, 69
Thrombocytopenia, 57
TMN stages, 22
Traditional Chinese Medicine (TCM), 59, 82, 118, 120, 127, 128, 129
Transcendental meditation, 140
Trypsin, 18
Tumors, sizes of, 22. *See also* Cancer

U

Ultrasound, 15
Urine, changes in color of, 8

V

VHL (Von Hippel–Lindau) gene, 27
Vincristine, 123
Vinorelbine, 123
Visualization, 142–43
Vitamins
  A, 97
  B1, 87–88
  B12, 88
  C, 88–89, 95, 96, 97, 99, 104, 111
  D, 89–91
  E, 97, 99, 111
  folic acid, 78–79
  K, 99
  multi-, 83–86
Vomiting, 8, 56, 80, 116, 121

W

Water, 112
Weight loss, 8
Whipple procedure, 39, 40–44, 45

Y

Yoga, 143–44

Z

Zinc, 99, 111